THE MAKING OF A PHYSICIAN

SHELDON COHEN M.D. FACP

Dedicated to

THE LOVES OF MY LIFE

Betty

Gail, Paul

Amanda, Megan, Carly, Alexa, Ethan, Emily, Derek, Rylie

BIOGRAPHICAL SKETCH

A graduate of the University Of Illinois College Of Medicine, the author has practiced internal medicine, served as a medical director of the Alexian Brother's Medical Center of Northwest Suburban Chicago and as medical director of two managed care organizations: Cigna Healthplan of Illinois and Humanicare Plus of Illinois. The author taught internal medicine and physical diagnosis to medical students from Loyola University Stritch School of Medicine and the Chicago Medical School, served as a consultant for Joint Commission Resources of the Joint Commission on Accreditation of Healthcare Organizations, did quality consultations at hospitals in the United States, Rio de Janeiro, Brazil, Copenhagen, Denmark, and served as a consultant to the Ministry of Health in Ukraine assisting them in the development of a hospital accrediting body. The author lectures to lay audiences on Risk Factor Analysis, Early Detection and Prevention, Symptoms Never to Ignore, The Prevention of Medical Errors, How to Take Charge of Your Own Healthcare, The Perfect Prescription, Hormones nerves and stress and other topics of a medical nature.

Dr. Cohen is the author of eighteen books.

TABLE OF CONTENTS

CHAPTER 1
PROLOGUE

I have decided to write an autobiography. Am I nationally or internationally famous? The answer is no, so who would care? Nobody, I'm sure. Being curious all my life about my ancestors, I've always wished I had more details about my grandparents, great grandparents and great-great grandparent's lives. I try to learn all I can from living relatives, but all I've been able to glean is very little or nothing at all because my interest peaked too late in life and there was no one left to query. Therefore, I decided I would spare my children, grandchildren and great grandchildren that same frustration…if they should ever have it. Why do I have it? I don't know except that I have become a writer (?) in my old age and have written many books as a way of keeping my aging brain intact. I can only hope that strategy is effective, but so far, it seems to be working; as I will soon be 83 years of age and still write. Notice there is no comment about the writing quality, which is not for me to say. I am confident, however, that my writing improves with time, practice and study. That opinion is mine and mine alone, so I continue to do my thing unencumbered by critical and professional comment. It is the best hobby I have ever embraced and I hope to continue it until I can no longer type or write.

Thinking it over, the best and most logical place to start this autobiography would be with the first memory of my life, so here goes.

The one thing I notice as I move further into seniority is the crispness of past memories. Now that I have time to think about the past—my mind not occupied by immediate work, home problems and challenges, it is incredible to me how some of those old memories parade through my consciousness like a three-dimensional color movie.

Do you recall your first memory? How old were you? Is it as distinct to you as mine is to me? I see it in my mind's eye as if it happened yesterday. I remember the exact location. I was sitting on the second floor outside porch of a two flat on Sacramento Boulevard, a block or two north of Augusta Boulevard, a middle-class neighborhood on the near-northwest side of Chicago of mixed ethnic heritage principally Jewish first or second-generation refugees from Eastern Europe and Polish Catholics who lived together in sort of an uneasy truce. My mother was either sitting next to me, or I was sitting on her lap, possibly both. I was able to look over the cement and brick-topped guardrail, and strangely enough, I still feel the excitement I felt as I watched a parade marching through Humboldt Park across the street. I was three years old, so it had to be 1933, a crucial year in world history.

Roosevelt started his New Deal, a social and economic program geared to get the country out of the Depression, which started the end of 1929 about a month before I was born on November 16. In 1933, Hitler became German chancellor and assumed total control of Germany with all that would portend for the world the next twenty-two years. Hitler's National Socialistic Deutcher Arbeiter Partie (National Socialist German Worker's Party), or Nazis for short, opened Dachau concentration Camp, the first of many to come. Japan left the League of Nations. The United States repealed prohibition, created The Tennessee Valley Authority and completed Hoover Dam. Morgan Thomas Hunt of the California Institute of Technology won the Nobel Prize in Physiology or Medicine "for his discoveries concerning the role played by the chromosome in heredity." Erwin Schrodinger of Berlin University and Paul Adrien Maurice Dirac of Cambridge University won the Nobel

Prize in Physics for their work clarifying Quantum Mechanics.

The world embarked upon changes for good and evil.

As I sat on that front porch and looked over the railing, soldiers marched on a diagonal street cutting through the park across from my home. They were dressed in what I would later recognize as World War I uniforms. I recall the ankle to knee khaki wrap that was such a distinctive part of the "doughboy's" uniform. The troops in the front row carried American flags. I suspect that I was watching a Fourth of July parade. I remember that the day was clear and warm. I can even remember gazing at my mother who was watching me as I manifested the excitement of the moment. The expression on her face is still clear in my mind. Now I would interpret it is an expression of the love of a mother for her child. The only thing I'm not sure about watching the parade is if a marching band played Fourth of July songs. I think they did, but it was the visual presentation rather than the auditory one that imprinted on my mind forever.

And that was my first memory, a memory that I cherish because circumstances were to develop in the future that would change that relationship between a mother and her son almost forever, but that is for later on in my story.

I often wondered how a simple event like that remains so vivid. On that day and at that time, under whatever conditions, the visual experience remains a part of my cerebral circuitry and has occupied a prominent place ever since. What were the physiological and other conditions at the time that allowed the imprinting of such a long lasting memory?

Whenever I ask friends to tell me about their first memory, they usually draw a blank. There is one exception to this, and that is a cousin of mine, Harvey, who is certain he remembers passing through the birth canal.

We all thought he was nuts, of course. "It's a dream," we said. However, later in life I read a report of a number of people who claim to remember their birth. Therefore, I prefer to lump my cousin in with this unusual group of people and accept that such a memory may be feasible. After all, no one can prove the converse.

One would think that a first memory involving a military parade would portend a military career for me, but I only spent two years in the army (during peacetime in the United States) and that is also a story for later on in my tale. However, I'm getting ahead of myself.

My maternal grandmother arrived in the United States in February of 1904 with my three-month-old future mother-to-be. Like all the other third-class immigrants of the time, when they landed in New York, they were required to pass through Ellis Island. They first settled in Rochester New York and later moved to Chicago. About twenty-five years later I was born on November 16, 1929 at Mount Sinai hospital, Chicago Illinois, a month after the great stock market crash that heralded the onset of the great Depression creating some of the economic conditions that would lead inevitably to the amazing history of the 1930's, the decade that paved the way to World War II.

CHAPTER 2
FAMILY HISTORY

My next memories occurred two years later. I was five years old and living in another apartment. Whereas I had lived on the second floor of the two flat with the cement and brick outdoor porch, I now lived on the second floor of another two flat (without a cement and brick porch). This new residence was two blocks further South on the same street—867 N. Sacramento Boulevard, Chicago, Illinois.

Only now, there was no father in the house. He left. There was no difference as far as my memory is concerned, for I have never had a recollection of a father in the house, and the only memory of my mother until I was five years old was the parade episode. Apparently, when I was a toddler, my mother fell mentally ill and spent a considerable amount of time in a "sanitarium." She often spoke about it later and mentioned her psychiatrist—Dr. Schoolman (sp?)—whose son I would later get to meet as a young adult while taking a math elective in medical school.

None of this registered in my brain, of course. My father was no longer with me, and during my mother's absence, maternal grandparents cared for me. My grandmother, who I called Bobby, a child's distorted Yiddish bubby, or grandmother, would become a great influence in my life. In essence, she served as a second mother. Her name was Anna Tepper and my grandfather's name was Sam. They served as substitute parents for me and provided me with loving care that I otherwise would have missed—and who knows what impact that would have had on my life.

My mother told me that once when she returned from the hospital, "You wouldn't come to me because you forgot who I was." She said these words with a sad expression that I remember to this day. At the time, I was standing in the dining room of my apartment and those words are a memory I will never forget, because, as young as I may have been, I felt how deeply that experience would affect any mother. It made me very sad, and I remember somehow feeling responsible.

My maternal grandmother and grandfather came from the Pale of Settlement, an area under Russian control. Specifically their hometown was Tiktin (Yiddish) Tykocin (Polish), a small town on the river Narew in northeast Poland. My maternal grandmother's name was Rosenovich. My maternal grandfather's name was Tepperovitch, subsequently Americanized to Tepper when they came to the United States through Ellis Island. The same is true of my paternal grandparents. Their name was Tombach (sp?), changed to Cohen when they arrived in the United States on passage through Ellis Island. There are three versions of this name change. 1. An Ellis Island clerk gave my grandfather the name Cohen, because he looked Jewish (a reflection of my grandfather's beard and heritage), 2. My grandfather changed his name to Cohen in order to get a "good American name," or 3. He changed his name as a reflection of his pride over the fact that he was descended from the first priestly tribe of ancient Israel, the Kohanim. I never learned which version was correct. Many years later, a man who I have confidence in told me that Ellis Island employees never gave immigrants a name. At this time, it would be appropriate to mention that my grandfather followed my grandmother and my infant mother to the United States. He was in the Czar's army, an army in which Jews could never be an officer, and in which Jews suffered persecution. Many years later, my cousin (my grandfather's son's daughter), told me that her father told her that my grandfather deserted the Czar's army, was captured by a Russian guard who said, "Let the young man go, his family is already in the United States." I have to wonder, if caught by another guard whether he would have suffered the fate of most deserters during wartime (Russo-Japanese war).

Why did my grandparents leave? Some history will be informative. It was in 1772 that Russia, Austria, and Prussia divided Poland in three stages over a period of twenty-seven years and my ancestors in Poland found themselves part of Russia. These partitions resulted in Russia assimilating several million Jews within their boundary. Most of these Jews comprised the middle class between the nobility and the peasantry of Russia.

At first, the Russian government tried to ignore them even though it was against government policy to have them within their borders, but eventually the government found them useful as they blamed the Jews for the untenable economic position of the peasants. As a result, the condition of the Jews became precarious, and the officials subjected them to onerous laws with ever-increasing restrictions.

The "Pale of Settlement" was the name of the entire landmass within which the Czar required Polish and other Eastern European Jews to live. As time went on, the geographic boundaries of the Pale would change and the living restrictions lifted for certain Jews who worked in some vital occupations, such as artisans, physicians, wealthy merchants, or graduates of universities; these were rare. The population of the Pale increased to almost five million by nineteen hundred.

In 1843, Nicholas I was Czar of Russia. He characterized the Jews as "the leeches of the country." He had instituted one of the most onerous laws in Jewish history when, in 1827, he decreed that once a Jew reached the age of twelve, he was required to serve in the Russian army for twenty-five years. At twelve, the authorities sent Jewish recruits to the same schools as the Russian soldier's sons. The purpose was simple. While serving in the military, a Jew had to convert or die.

In general, they had to endure ill treatment by their officers, and religious authorities subjected them to various tortures in order to accept baptism. Awakened in the middle of the night and compelled to kneel until they accepted conversion or collapse, their tormentors gave them high salt meals with no water, beat and tortured them and it was the rare recruit who was able to hang on to his faith.

Jewish communities received a quota of Jewish twelve-year-olds to supply to the military. This quota was a certain number of conscripts per each thousand males. Who would go? Who would not go? In some areas, authorities forced children of the poorest Jews into service. Influential Jewish leaders assigned to this task hired "khapers" to fill the quota. In essence, these hired men were salaried kidnapers.

Upon entering the military, Jewish children lived in barracks called cantonments and as a result, the authorities named them cantonists.

My maternal grandparents first settled in Rochester, New York and then Chicago, Illinois where my maternal grandfather went to work for his wealthy brother-in-law, a prominent bakery owner and investor named Sam Rosen who became a master baker at the age of twelve following a three-year apprenticeship in Germany. In the thirties, I can remember my grandfather's salary of thirty-five dollars a week, and the rent on Sacramento Boulevard of thirty dollars per month. On that income, he raised three daughters and one son.

My father was also born in Tiktin four years before my mother. His parents and my mother's parents knew each other in the old country. My father's mother died aged twenty-six. I've heard two versions as to the cause of death: childbirth or pneumonia. I suspect the former is more accurate, but I'm not certain. Regardless, my paternal grandfather became a widower, and in time married a sixteen-year-old girl (my future step-grandmother) and immigrated to the United States—in 1904. This was most fortunate for my step grandmother because during World War II her twelve brothers and sisters who remained in Poland were lost in the Holocaust. I learned about this as a teen, after WWII, when I was at a cousin club meeting that my father's family would hold on a regular basis. My step-grandmother told me the story. It had an impact, because it remains as a vivid memory in my mind; one of those memories where the expression on my step grandmother's face etched in my mind as was my mother's memory on the porch overlooking Humboldt Park.

My father, as was the custom of the time in immigrant Jewish homes, had a fourth grade education—enough to learn the rudiments of reading and writing and 'rithmetic—and then proceeded to learn a trade—plumbing.

My maternal grandfather also told me that he knew my father's family in the 'old country,' and when my father's mother died, "I picked up your father and put him on my lap. He was about four or five years old. I wiped his nose and told him you see, Ben, even God can make a mistake."

This is the background of my grandparents who fled Eastern Europe, came to this country and enjoyed the freedoms they could never have in The Pale. It took many years for them to stop looking over their shoulder. They raised their children and assimilated as United States citizens. They learned English, but spoke Yiddish in the home. They spoke with me in Yiddish, and I would answer in English. I lived with them until I went away to college. They played a major role in whatever I was able to achieve in life.

My mother tells me, after her divorce, "That when I was going to marry your father, grandpa was real happy.

I think I married him because your grandfather wanted it. I don't think I ever loved him."

But my mother's illness was more than my grandfather could cope with. He could not comprehend the concept of mental illness. My mother's depression was bad enough, but her failure to touch anything, apparently out of fear of spreading the "contamination" she picked up in the "sanitarium," drove him to distraction and resulted in her alienation from much of the family. As I grew up, I must confess I too found it difficult to be able to cope. I couldn't understand why she only touched objects in the home with paper, would never touch me, and why, if I touched her, I had to wash my hands. She claimed that while in the sanitarium "a flame went out of my body. They took my soul. I have no soul." This thinking and behavior persisted all her adult life, associated with bouts of depression, but never any more hallucinatory symptoms. In my mother's late eighties, she slowly lapsed into mild senility and forgetfulness ("you're my son?"). Her old mental symptoms resolved and finally I was able to hug her and kiss her cheek and hold her hand without her panicking; and I did not have to wash my hands or lips. It felt good.

She died at age 92 while holding my hand, something she would never allow in her younger years. While grasping her hand in mine I fell asleep in the chair. When I awakened, she was gone. I had the thought that she put me to sleep so I would not see her die. My family, the medical profession, nor I, had never been able to help her. Only time and an altered aging brain healed her mind. I am hopeful this meant that God returned her soul before she died, for during life her biggest fear was dying without a soul. "How could you die without a soul?" she would ask.

In spite of it, all she managed to function normally away from home. She worked for famous Chicago lawyers, performed as the Parent Teacher's Association secretary for many years, typed 100 plus words a minute and played Dark town Stutter's Ball on the piano. The LaSalle street lawyers she worked for praised her as an unlicensed attorney. And she was able to accomplish this after only two years of high school. "Why only two years?" I asked. "Because most of my friends were standing in the two year line during registration, so that's where I went." She led her class academically. Her brother, a physician, marveled at her brilliance. He looked forward to the grammatically perfect letters he received from her during World War II while he served as a physician in the army. She excelled in her own way in spite of the tremendous odds and misunderstanding of the time levied against her. I owe her much. She was an example of what psychologically challenged people could accomplish. No one ever diagnosed her with a label other than depression, but the few hallucinatory bouts as a young woman makes me wonder if she did have a schizoaffective disorder. I didn't know enough then—and I still don't—to come to a firm psychiatric diagnosis.

CHAPTER 3
EARLY DAYS

I never felt the great depression of the 1930's as many American citizens did. We were lucky. My great-uncle, Sam Rosen, who, as mentioned, owned the bakery on Division Street in Chicago and provided steady employment for his sister's husband (my grandfather), assured my family of a steady and stable income of thirty-five dollars a week. On this income, my grandfather raised his family, a wife, three daughters and one son, in a three bedroom flat on Sacramento Blvd. Much later in life, I learned that Sam Rosen, when a nine-year-old boy in Poland, spent time in Germany as a baker's apprentice, worked his way up to a full baker, and by 18 years of age emigrated to the United States, first living in New York, where I heard rumors to the extent that he became a Union organizer, had difficulties with "the mob" and fled to Chicago where he earned his fortune becoming a multi-millionaire, especially famous for his "Rosen's Rye Bread," which surrounded every corned beef sandwich made in the city of Chicago and the mid-west for decades.

As a young boy in the 1930's, my memories of the depression were a series of letters, WPA, CCC, plus other letters that referred to Roosevelt's New Deal, our presidents ambitious effort to lift the country out of the major depression that threatened not only the United States, but also spread its deadly tentacles to the rest of the world playing no small part in events leading to the conditions that had an influence on the development of World War II with all its horrific consequences.

Roosevelt took the bulls by the horn and instituted the New Deal, his effort to give the federal government more responsibility for the economic welfare of the people. States declared a moratorium on bank withdrawals to prevent depositors from withdrawing their funds thus bankrupting the banks, but Roosevelt declared a four-day banking holiday and attested to the fact that the banks were sound, restoring confidence and subsequently insured deposits through the Federal Deposit Insurance Corporation FDIC. Roosevelt also established agencies to provide government-sponsored work for the unemployed developing special projects to provide employment for artists, writers, musicians and actors through the Works Project Administration (WPA), initials I was familiar with as one of my friend's father was an unemployed artist who found employment with the WPA. There was also the Public Works Administration (PWA) employing men aged 18 to 25 through the Civilian Conservation Corps (CCC) for forest work, construction of highways, dams, buildings and other conservation projects..

During the depression, prices and wages fell. To stem this disaster, Roosevelt developed the National Industrial Recovery Act that promoted the cooperation of labor and management in setting prices, wages and hours worked and gave all employees the right to join unions. Roosevelt also put crop reduction measures in place to reduce farm surpluses, which were responsible for the low prices. Other projects included the Tennessee Valley Authority to develop an underdeveloped area of the country, the Security and Exchange Commission to regulate the stock market and the Social Security Act providing for unemployment insurance and old age pensions.

The country reelected Roosevelt for an unprecedented third term.

I have several memories when I was five years old. The most important one was the decision to become a physician. I attribute this interest to my uncle, my mother's brother, Sidney, who, in 1935, was a second year medical student at the University of Illinois. By this time, my father and mother had separated, and my mother and I moved in with my grandparents. I can remember my uncle sitting at the dining room table peering through a microscope. He would pick me up and put me on his lap, and point out a world of bacteria, blood cells, and different body tissues. I can remember the fascination I felt, etching in my mind the path as a future doctor. My uncle became the father figure that I never had, and I remain grateful to his memory. My own father finally divorced my mother when I was ten. He would pick me up on Saturdays, and would spend the day with me until I became a teenager and then I would visit him on Saturdays in his plumbing shop where he would put me to work. I soon learned the name of every piece of plumbing apparatus available. When I was eighteen years of age, he moved to California with his young wife, Shirley.

My uncle became a physician in 1938. He served an internship for two years at Cook County Hospital, Chicago, worked for a short time in Parsons, Kansas where he found his future wife. Then he spent six years in the army medical corps during World War II serving in both the Pacific and European theatre of operations. The only thing I ever heard him say about his experience was, "Those Japanese pilots flew so low I could see the expression on their faces." He had a long and illustrious career as a California obstetrician and gynecologist. Without my realizing it, I believe he taught me how to set a goal at this time in my life.

My mother's youngest sister Harriet married Sam Siegel, and he fought in the Battle of the Bulge. My mother's other sister, Rose, won a Chicago Charleston dance contest during the roaring twenties and married Leo Manhoff who was too old to serve in World War II. These two uncles also served somewhat as a father figure for me. I was fortunate to have such a loving family to provide support.

I have very few memories of kindergarten, but the one that stands out is my first day of school. I met my teacher, Miss Kimble. She had snow-white hair, and looked like everyone's grandmother. One of my class-mates announced that he had to go to the washroom, so Miss Kimble unbuttoned his union suit in the rear. He promptly let it fall and walked to the bathroom with his buttocks exposed. We all laughed. I can still see him walking as vividly as I remember the parading soldiers.

I never got to the first semester of first grade. In-stead, I suffered a series of contagious diseases. My mother tells me I had whooping cough, followed by measles, and finally German measles and mumps. In those days, the order was to quarantine, so I spent the entire first semester in bed.

It's strange, but the next episode, perhaps of critical importance in my life, is only vaguely present in my memory. The first semester of the first grade served to set the foundation for basic reading. My mother knew this, so she purchased a blackboard and chalk, and while I was in bed, she taught me how to read...a practitioner of "home schooling" before its time. I vaguely remem-ber the blackboard on an easel and my mother standing beside the bed lecturing to me. When she spoke of the experience, she told me how rapidly I learned all the letters and words. I think she used a self-invented system of phonics long before it became popular. Of course, I never realized the loving and critical importance of this action.

Since I missed the first semester of the first grade, my mother brought me to school to meet my second se-mester first grade teacher, Miss DiMatta. I remember her appearance: short, thin, coal black hair, glasses, and a superior air. She told my mother that even though I missed the first semester, and therefore did not learn to read, she would pass me onto the second semester, but put me in the "slow group" and hope I would be able to catch up.

"Oh no,"` my mother said, "I taught him how to read. He doesn't need to be in the slow group."

Miss DiMatta was incredulous, and said she couldn't do that because I had missed the entire semester, but my mother insisted that I they give me a book and test me on the spot. The principle, Mr. Garret Rickard, agreed. How did I ever remember that name? Anyhow, I read the book with ease and joined the second semester advanced group. I can still remember the upstaged look on Miss DiMatta's face. I was worried about it, but I didn't know why. Things must have worked out because I have no further recollection of the first grade.

I lived almost a mile from LaFayette Grade School. In kindergarten and first grade, my mother walked me there every day. This meant four round trip walks. We never could afford a car, and even if we could, it was rare in those days to have women drivers. She brought me to school in the morning, walked back home, picked me up at school for lunch at home (there were no school lunches then—or busses), brought me back to school after lunch, came back home, picked me up after school and walked back home with me. I don't remember how long it took me to protest that "I could do it myself," but eventually I did.

CHAPTER 4
GRADE SCHOOL

The first grade must have been good for I became an avid reader. Since I knew what direction my life would take, I spent my spare time reading books about the human body, biology, physiology, health, hygiene, science in general. My personal private life was good, but my home life became an environment I needed to conceal from friends. There were constant verbal battles between my mother and her parents and sisters. "They don't know what I'm going through," my mother would say. Apparently, she thought her aberrant behavior was borne of absolute necessity. "Someday people will know I was right." My uncle, who by now was involved in WWII, left with the statement to the family that "if Sheldon had to live through those family battles, he would probably end up in a straight jacket."

The battles became so verbally abusive that I would expect to come home in the middle of a fight. So, if I ever would arrive home with friends I would always run ahead of them and fly up the stairs to be able to quiet things down before my friends would arrive. It was uncomfortable and difficult and I was always fearful of having a friend over.

As best as I knew I was the only one of my friends who had divorced parents. In those days, divorce was a rare phenomenon. It made me feel different, and I lived with that knowledge, but my mechanism of handling it was to ignore that it was reality. If people spoke of it, I left the room or changed the subject. I am sure that current thinking would be totally against such an approach, but I think it worked for me. I can recall my cousin Harvey, dumbfounded by my pretense, say, "God, is he dumb." I ignored that comment by pretending I never heard it. Harvey's sister, Sheila, was my good friend and youthful playmate as was Marshall, my aunt Rose's son.

Although my upbringing and parental relationship was different from my friends and relatives, I had the support of an extended family. In those days, families lived in close proximity and provided mutual support for each other. On one block of Sacramento Boulevard, I had my mother, grandparents, all my aunts, uncles and an assorted collection of cousins.

So this is the way I grew up, an emotional loner, but finding the strength to resolve problems by myself. I did very well in school, but thought that the more I knew about the human body, the greater would be my chance of becoming a doctor, so I concentrated on subjects I thought necessary, but made an error by ignoring two subjects I disliked—math and English. "I don't need math. I can talk so why worry about these grammar details." Even if someone had told me I was wrong, I would have probably ignored that sound advice. I focused on my scientific interest. It was almost a fatal mistake—but more later.

CHAPTER 5
MORE GRADE SCHOOL

Sacramento Boulevard was strictly a residential street. Division Street was a mile away and was mostly commercial. There was a Walgreen's drug store on the corner of Division and California where my mother would often take me for a thick malted milk with two cookies if I remember correctly. On Saturday, she would often take my cousins and me to a movie at the Division Theatre on Division Street that featured the weekly serial, Flash Gordon. For twenty-five cents (?), you saw the serial and the feature film and received some dishes. Going every week guaranteed that you would get the entire collection of chinaware.

I remember my fifth grade teacher very well. Her name was Miss Ryan. She was short and very pretty to the perception of a ten-year-old boy, and I think I was the "teacher's pet." I distinctly remember one episode, because I lied to her. It was the first time I can ever remember telling a fib.

Miss Ryan gave the fifth grade class an assignment. She wanted us to write an essay titled "The Two Greatest Inventions in the History of the World." I wracked my brains and came up blank. However, through an amazing coincidence, I happened to have a science book that I planned to read. One of the chapters titled "The World's Two Greatest Inventions" opened my eyes and I proceeded to digest every word. According to the book, the two inventions that had the greatest impact on world history were <u>language</u> and the <u>wheel</u>. I had my essay.

The day after we handed in the assignment Miss Ryan took me aside and said, "Sheldon, where did you get your greatest inventions idea?"

"Uhh…I just thought of it," I said in a matter of fact way. Then I looked at Miss Ryan's face to see the effect.

She nodded her head, and I interpreted the expression on her face to be one of amazement that a ten-year-old boy should have such a profound understanding of the concepts that could so expand civilization and world progress. At least that's what I thought her expression meant at the time. More than likely, her thoughts were—yeah, right, you little fibber.

There it was. I told a fib with the ulterior motive of wanting my teacher to think that I was this smart, deep thinking, little kid. I believe I remember this episode so vividly because of the lie I told. I knew I was doing wrong.

Another major memory I have of grade school was in the sixth grade in 1941. Upper grade children went to the auditorium. There was a large radio on the stage and we all heard Franklin Delano Roosevelt give his famous days of infamy speech to announce the entry of the United States into World War II after the Japanese attack on Pearl Harbor. Everyone remembers where he was that fateful day. I had been to a Chicago Bears football game. When I arrived back home I found my grandmother crying. She told me that the Japanese attacked the country and we would be at war. She had a personal reason to cry. Her son was already in the army medical corp. In fact, the army assigned him to a troop ship heading for the Philippines some months prior, but they ordered him off the ship at the last minute and replaced him by an unmarried physician. He had married his Kansas sweetheart by that time. Who knows if he would have survived the Bataan Death March, or if his replacement did?

Lafayette grade school provided me with many pleasurable memories. My mother, aunts and uncles preceded me there. There were no middle schools. One went from kindergarten to eighth grade in grammar school and then four years of high school.

My social life started in eighth grade. At age thirteen, we had a flurry of parties. A large group of girls and boys would get together to celebrate birthdays and other occasions at various homes (never mine) and about the only memory I have of these events was the great game we played—spin the bottle. With luck, my bottle would end up pointing to Eleanor. At that point you would leave the circle, go into another room (usually the bedroom), and collect your reward—a kiss. Where were the parents I wonder? I never saw Eleanor after the eighth grade, but I think she was my first female interest. Eleanor and spin the bottle would have to do for a very long time. My high school and college career saw no great advance in this realm of activity.

Age thirteen saw another advance, however, in my maturation process. The Bar Mitzvah ceremony. I became a man. We had a synagogue service and a dinner at the Midwest Athletic club with family and friends. This put my mother and father in the same room together, always an uncomfortable time for me.

Since I was a Kohen, the synagogue looked forward to this event, for now they would have a priestly descendent to bless the congregation. This meant that I would be involved in the prayer ritual. Since this was an orthodox synagogue, the principles washed my feet and then I would go up on the stage in front of the Torah and before the congregation. As instructed, I positioned the back of my hands in front of my face with thumbs touching and second and third fingers separated from the fourth and fifth fingers. A large prayer shawl covered my upper body, head, face and hands. The purpose of this was to keep my face hidden from the congregants, for while I chanted the prayer anyone who looked at my face would die on the spot, so they told me. While I was on the stage, I was able to look downward and see the floor immediately in front of the stage. Marching there were my classmates who looked up at me and viewed my face. After the ceremony they said, "We looked right in your face and we're still alive." This was a great relief, for the last thing I wanted was to be responsible for the premature demise of my friends.

Now that I was a "man," I started going to the synagogue with my grandfather every Saturday. After services, the rabbi asked me to escort one of the older parishioners home. He was very short, stooped over, had a long snow-white beard, lived two blocks away, and the trip took one half-hour. He was 103 years old and his method of locomotion was a very slow shuffle. One-hundred and three years old in 1943 meant he was born in 1840, twenty-one years before the Civil War.

I do not remember how many times I made that walk, but I do remember slowly fading out of Saturday services.

Grammar school graduation was another event bringing my mother and father together. The good news was that they would be sitting in the audience, not together, of course, and I would be on the stage. One part of the program was to be a short play and I hoped to get a role. I did not, but they assigned me the task of taking the chairs off the stage after the band finished a few patriotic pieces. That made my part in the graduation ceremony a member of the stage labor force, while my classmates either played their instruments or had an opportunity to demonstrate their theatrical skills. Although my performance in front of my parents was, to say the least, unimpressive, I received my diploma (still hanging on my wall) and would soon move on to Tuley High School.

What else did I do my first thirteen years?

There was a large park across the street from where I lived, and across that park was a large playground and swimming pool. We would spend almost every day in summer swimming in that pool. You would wait on a long group of benches to get your turn for a one-hour swim. It was great exercise and I became a credible swimmer. I actually saved one drowning boy's life as he sunk and could not ascend. I had completely forgotten this episode, only to be reminded of it at a fifty-year high school reunion when the boy I saved reminded the class of what I had done when he thanked me for "still being here due to Sheldon."

Also, about a mile from my home on Division Street there was the Deborah Boy's Club where club members held meetings, played ping pong and basketball. The basketball court was on the second floor and it had a low ceiling necessitating learning how to shoot the basketball in a straight trajectory—no arch. A no arch shot labeled one as a player who learned his craft at Deborah Boy's Club.

About a mile from the house, in Humboldt Park, there were multiple tennis courts. With a three-dollar tennis racquet, purchased from Walgreen's by my mother, I learned how to play with fellow friends all learning together from scratch with no instruction except from the older players.

Speaking of Walgreen's, this reminds me of what could have been the start of a criminal career. At aged thirteen, I started taking trumpet lessons. I would take the streetcar to downtown Chicago's Wabash Street, take my lesson, go downstairs to the corner Walgreen's and buy a malted milk. Then I would take a five-cent streetcar ride back home. On one occasion, I took my lesson, went to Walgreen's, enjoyed my malted milk and reached into my pocket to retrieve money to pay the bill. Lo and behold, all I had was five cents for carfare home. What was I to do? In a panic, I strolled around the store, up and down the aisles, and then headed past the cashier for the door—and I just walked out. Now I am ashamed to say that that was so easy that I did it four more times until my conscience got the better of me. Now as I write this, I have decided to send them payment—belatedly, but better late than never. So thirty-five times five is equal to one dollar and seventy-five cents, times, figure five percent interest for about sixty-four years, equals whatever. Once I can pull out my calculator and figure it out I will send the money to Walgreen's and finally assuage my conscience. Better late then never.

After grade school I moved on to Tuley High School, where again, my mother and aunts and uncles had preceded me. Today, the high school is a grammar school. A new high school, built at a location several blocks away and named Roberto Clemente High School, is a reflection of the neighborhood's new ethnic heritage. The old Tuley High School became a grade school.

CHAPTER 6
HIGH SCHOOL

I remember my first day in high school. I arrived forty minutes late. My grandmother awakened me at the wrong time. I think I cried. I know I was distraught. My poor grandmother! The high school was two miles away and I had to take a streetcar ride to get there—if I didn't walk. I arrived late and watched uncomfortably as the teacher stared me into my seat. Freshman students of Tuley high school attended a separate school called Sabin. The last three years we transferred to Tuley, the school where my mother and all my aunts and uncles attended.

PAUSE

At this point in the book, please be advised that the pause (above) represents five years. Yes, it is five years later and I have not written a word for five years. I've been involved with other books, but neglected this one and almost forgot about it. But now that I have no other books in mind, and since I've reached the age of eighty-two, I thought I would make an effort to make a change or two and complete this book before I reach the age of eighty-five (if I do) where statistics tell me that I have a fifty-fifty chance of evolving into Alzheimer's disease. So here I go…before it's too late…

To reiterate (I mentioned this before), I started high school in 1943 while World War II was raging on. On Pearl Harbor day, Sunday, December 7, 1941, as a twelve-year-old in grade school, I attended a Chicago Bear's football game at Wrigley Field. When I arrived home, I found my grandmother crying. She told me that we were at war. Her tears were justified; her son, my uncle, Sidney, was already in the United States Army medical Corps. There was a doctor draft at the time, something I would learn about very directly years later. My uncle served a total of six years during which he spent time in the Pacific theater (Aleutian Islands) and the European theater of operations, as I've already mentioned. Thankfully, he returned home after the war to resume his medical career. Other members of my family that fought in the war were my uncle, Sam Siegel, who fought at the battle of the bulge and two cousins, Russell and Jay Topper who fought in Europe as tankers with George Patton as best as I can remember. They all returned safely. During wartime, I busied myself as a student who participated in scrap and paper drives, "for the war effort." I followed the course of the war religiously via radio, the newspapers and a one-hour news theater once per week when I went downtown to take my trumpet lesson. I think I knew every island hopping battle fought in the Pacific as well as following the European battles.

I have very little remembrance of my first year at Tuley high school spent at Sabin. I was a good student getting mostly S's and some E's in a system where S stood for superior, or A; E stood for Excellent or B; G stood for good, or C. The second year is when most activities started. I will divide them into three categories: academic, social and athletic.

Academically I did well ending up near the top of my class behind the two "biggest brains" Nick and George. Nick became an attorney and George, I believe, became a teacher and school principal. I realize that all the reading I had done as a pre-teen; the human body, medical history "Rats, Lice and History" by Hans Zinnser, etc, trained my brain in the memorization of facts, but my dislike of mathematical subjects (just getting by with good grades) and only doing the minimum of work would come to haunt me later in college. Although adults told me of math's importance, I paid no attention to the wisdom of elders. After all, who knows more than a thirteen-year-old? Unfortunately, I had to get older to realize this almost fatal mistake (more when the book takes us to the college years). I took Latin as a foreign language. After all, didn't doctors speak and write prescriptions in Latin?

As you can see, I missed the wisdom of my uncle, away in the Aleutian Islands where "I could see the Japanese pilots smiling in their cockpits."

Socially, as regards the opposite sex, a few paragraphs should about do it for my four years of high school. I was sixteen and madly in love, we dated a few times and I took her to the junior prom. In addition, we went to the Daily News relays (an annual track and field meet) at the Chicago Stadium. This was the first time she witnessed track and field events. Amazed, she asked me, "What is that guy doing with the long pole?" I finally kissed her good night after the fourth or fifth date (only after asking permission) and subsequently learned that her father was an active member of the Communist Party. On one date, I picked her up at the Abraham Lincoln School in downtown Chicago (The Loop) and she asked me to sign my name on a guest (?) register. Ten years later when I filled out an application for the doctor draft (compulsory two years of military service), one of the questions was… have you ever been a member of one of the following subversive organizations? There it was…the Abraham Lincoln School.

I don't remember the details about how the relationship ended, but it did. I believe she lost interest in continuing to date me and I lost track of her, but a friend of mine married her younger sister and I learned that she married a Professor of Russian History at the University of Chicago.

The area where I grew up had its rough elements as I learned the hard way. Walking down Walton Street with two friends, Lee and Fred, a younger boy on a bicycle approached and his bicycle must have hit an impediment, because, if I remember correctly, he fell off. I made a comment that he apparently did not take kindly, and he pedaled off in haste only to return within minutes with a group of older boys. The bicycle rider pointed me out, most of the older boys surrounded me, told my two friends to step back and one of them let me know that he was going to "Beat the s--t out of me." Finding myself on the ground, arms and legs flailing in all directions, it soon became apparent to a surprised me that I was getting the best of him reflected by the massive amount of blood, from his nose, now all over my jacket. Since we were ruining the front yard of a neighbor, an adult man came out of his house, separated us and chased us away. My friends and I promptly left for our respective homes. I can still remember my shocked mother and grandmother when I entered the apartment and they saw the blood all over my jacket. "You should see the other guy," was my only comment.

This little episode made the neighborhood a difficult place to walk around, and sure enough, within one week, my friend Lee and I were in a candy store on Walton near Francisco. I was interested in purchasing a ten-cent comic book displayed in the front window when my friend Lee pointed out to me that our friends, including the one I had the altercation with, were standing outside the store staring at us through the window. Lee panicked, but that and the knowledge that I had already licked this guy gave me some misplaced courage to say, "Don't let them think you're scared." Then I walked outside the store, mingled between them while at the same time ignoring them and looking at the display in the front window while pointing out to the proprietor the comic book I wanted. I went back in the store, paid my ten cents, told Lee to act confident and follow me out of the store. They never touched us.

I soon began to envision myself as this heroic fellow working as a spy or a commando, landing on a dark beach in a clandestine attack.

If I only had the brains to save all those first edition comic books I purchased.

Another time, I attended a Tuley football game. The Second World War ended. The year was forty-six, possibly forty-seven. After the game, I was walking home, still near the stadium when someone struck me from behind causing me to lose my balance and fall to the ground. Without thinking, my spontaneous reaction was to say, "Who do you think you're pushing?" and as I looked up, I saw a group of older young men dressed in Navy uniforms. At the sound of my voice they stopped and one of them said, "Hey, there's the guy that said the Navy's full of s--t." With that, several of them attacked me, knocked me against a fence, threw me on the ground and began to pummel me unmercifully. That seemed to be lasting forever until, out of the corner of my eye, I could see two of my classmates running toward me, leap into the air, land feet first on the faces of my two assailants causing them to turn their attention away from me. Joe Greco and another friend of his started beating them without let-up. A Tuley assistant principal pulled me away and local police rushed upon the scene and ended the fight. I went home on the bus, hoping that this episode had ended.

I don't want the reader to get the impression that I attended a rough high school. In my experience, the above were the only violent episodes in four years. Tuley had an excellent reputation academically all through the twenties, thirties, and forties when my aunt Harriet used to walk to school with Saul Bellow, the future Nobel Prize winner in Literature.

Athletically, I involved myself in two sports. The three dollar tennis racket that my mother purchased for me, and the Humboldt Park practice routine playing pick-up games put me in good stead, for I made the team early and became number two singles my junior year. Not all Chicago high schools had tennis teams, but the suburban teams did have teams and they were the powerhouses of tennis in the Chicago area, a reflection of the wealthy suburbs where tennis courts graced back yards and wealthy suburbanites gave their children tennis lessons. We played against tennis teams from the city and the suburbs, and as number two singles, I won every match my junior year. My number one singles teammate, Bill, and I qualified as one of four Chicago tennis doubles teams to vie for the state championship, but the suburban team we played against, Riverside, defeated us in the first round, thanks to my sloppy play. As a reward for winning all my number two matches as a junior, Coach Tortorelli promoted me to number one singles my senior year. I promptly rewarded his insight by not winning a single match. Obviously, the level of competition at the number one single's level was a level or more above.

Basketball was the second and only other high school sport I participated in, a sport where I learned my craft at the Deborah Boy's Club on Division Street, the low ceiling, low arch required shot where I played almost daily pick-up games and where different teams competed in various tournaments. Enough of those games and, as some told me, natural athletic talent, made it possible for me to make the senior team. By senior team, I mean the team for boys five foot eight inches or taller as there was also a junior team for boys less than five feet eight. I worked my way up the ranks, so that by the time I became a senior, I was in the running for the starting first team. I remember at the time feeling that this decision would be the most important thing that could ever happen to me, but at the same time, I had a tendency to re-alize that it wasn't very important in the greater scheme of things, so I developed a philosophy of…do you really think this is so important? Would you feel like this twenty years from now when you could look back on this decision, which is bugging you so much right now? The answer is clearly no, so cool it…what happens, happens. I think this philosophical mind-set put me in good stead for other problems faced during the rest of my life.

However, the worry was for naught as Coach Tor-torelli picked me for the first team as a starting guard. The other guard was George Olyszewski, center was Joe Grabowski and the two forwards were Izzy Feldman and Kenneth Adalbert. As a starting guard, my job was to get defensive rebounds, disrupt fast breaks, help bring the ball down on offense, and guard the other team's high scorers. In this role, I did not score many baskets, but my teammates did. We won West Section and played for the City title. In the semi-final game against South Shore, I learned a lesson I will never forget.

South Shore had an All-State player named Jake Fendley. He would go on to be All- American at North-western University and play professional basketball. At six feet three, he was one of the taller players in the state with the agility and quickness of a cheetah. When Coach Tortorelli assigned me to guard him, telling me that we could win if I could stifle Jake, I had no idea what awaited me. It would be an awakening. In a basketball era when forty to thirty was a high scoring game, I held Fendley to…twenty-seven points in the first half where-upon Coach Tortorelli had enough of me, replacing me defensively with Joe Grabowski, six feet and seven inches, the tallest basketball player in the state, who fared no better guarding Jake and fouled out. Two ex-amples of Fendley's expertise served to quickly put me in my place and made me realize that there was another

level of basketball greatness that very few could reach—
and for sure, I was not one of those few. First, stationed
on defense at the free throw line in my best defensive
posture I waited as Fendley approached dribbling the
basketball. While thinking that he's not going to get by
me, he suddenly disappeared from my field of vision.
Where was he…I lost him, but I turned around and there
he was scoring two points with a simple lay-up. I did not
see him go past me on my left; I did not see him go past
me on my right. The only conclusion I could think of is
that he passed right through me—he had to be a ghost. I
broke out in a cold sweat. The second time, I was in the
same position on the free-throw line while Fendley again
dribbled toward me. I crouched, bouncing on my toes,
determined not to have a repeat of the first episode, only
this time instead of faking me out, he leaped up in the
air. What the hell is he doing, I thought, the basket is
way back there. And I watched as he floated in the air
toward the basket for another simple lay-up and two
more points. Anti-gravity, I could only conclude. The
man was superhuman. That was enough for Tortorelli
and I spent the rest of the game on the bench.

But for me, it was a humbling experience, for it in-
stantly dawned upon me that there was another level of
basketball expertise that I could not reach.

Thus ended my high school career; a good four
years with a fun-filled athletic experience, an inactive
social life and an interesting academic experience except
for English and math, two subjects I chose to deempha-
size as unimportant, although I can say that geometry
fascinated me. I was on my way to the University of Illinois.

CHAPTER 7
COLLEGE

In 1947 when I started at the University of Illinois, many World War II veterans entered college on the G.I. bill. The initials stood for Government Issue, and G.I. was the slang initials standing for any person who served in the military. This important bill made it possible to attend college for those who heretofore may not have been able to afford it. It remains as one of the most successful programs in United States history. The increased incoming student load forced universities to expand, and the University of Illinois, always located at Champaign-Urbana, Illinois, chose to expand by opening two satellite universities: Galesburg, Illinois in what I believe was an old veteran's hospital, and Chicago, Illinois located at Navy Pier, an old Chicago landmark jutting out onto Lake Michigan. The university reserved the Champaign-Urbana campus for mostly returning veterans and left the two satellites for high school graduates and those veterans who preferred to go there. I chose Galesburg and embarked on a train ride late at night with my mother and father at the station. Arriving at Galesburg very early in the morning when it was still dark, I took a cab to the university where they gave me a temporary cot. The next morning I started the sign-in process, took some exams and found that I had proficiencied out of two required freshman courses in the health and hygiene area undoubtedly a reflection of my extensive reading in such subjects. Too bad I did not do the same in math and English...as I would soon find out. The English course assigned to me was semantics and the math course was trigonometry. They would both give me fits and I would end up with two C's, an inauspicious beginning for a pre-med. Fortunately my other grades kept me in the running and I had no thoughts of giving up on becoming a doctor. A few Tuley graduates also attended Galesburg and I would meet many new friends who would remain so the rest of our lives.

We lived in a dormitory and slept on cots with an adjacent locker for our possessions. There were at least twenty of us in each dormitory, some of whom were World War II veterans. Other veterans occupied private rooms in an extended hallway leading to the dormitory portion. I grew up fast. It was not unusual to see veterans bring young women in their rooms and close the door. What were they doing in there, I wondered. The younger ones of us found out when we put our ears to the door.

I did manage to renew my athletic career with intramural basketball. Our dormitory team won the Galesburg basketball championship, and the selection committee appointed me captain of the all-star team. Put that in your pipe and smoke it, Jake!

By the end of the first year at Galesburg my grade point average in spite of the C's was still in the range of possibility for medical school and I vowed to strive on, but before returning to Galesburg an episode occurred that forced me to change schools. Now for that story.

My mother, grandmother and grandfather lived back home in the same location, 867 N. Sacramento Blvd. where I grew up. Before I left for Galesburg, my grandfather developed a cardiac problem, for which there was very little that could be done medically at that time. He developed 'heart block.'

By way of explanation, the heart is an amazing electrical machine, and each heartbeat of the ventricles starts by an electrical impulse that originates in the right atrium, prompts the atria to beat, then travels downwards and prompts the lower heart chambers, the ventricles, to beat pumping blood to the body. If scars from a heart attack disrupt this electrical pathway, the ventricles may not receive their electrical message. The logical question is to ask—then how do the ventricles beat? Yes, they do beat by virtue of an intrinsic rhythm that God, in his or her wisdom built in to the ventricles as a safety valve. This intrinsic rhythm, however, beats at a slower rate, and the rate can get slow enough to cause syncope (fainting spells). Currently, a patient exhibiting these symptoms would be fitted with a cardiac electronic pacemaker that will trigger a normal heart rate if it senses a heart rate below a preset limit. My grandfather, or any other patient of the time, would not have been able to take advantage of this advance, as there were no electronic pacemakers. Therefore, he was a laboratory for the natural course of this disease, which was to get a slower and slower heart rate making him prone to syncope, known as Stokes-Adams attacks. This is a sudden loss of consciousness because of a heart rate that has gotten too slow. My grandmother would hear a thump on the floor, and find my grandfather lying unconscious. His ventricles, in its intrinsic genius, would in time speed up enough for him to regain consciousness. When I returned from Galesburg for a visit on one occasion, my grandfather fell unconscious. I picked him up off the floor, carried him to the bedroom, and placed him on his back on the bed. I could not feel a pulse. I was about to tell my grandmother the bad news when I suddenly felt a pulse beat, so I kept on palpating his radial pulse and after what seemed like an eternity I felt another heartbeat. I kept counting and I felt one heart beat every six seconds for a heart rate of ten beats per minute. Finally, it sped up, and he regained consciousness.

In all the years I have practiced medicine, I never had a patient with a heartbeat as slow as when I was a teenager and had my first cardiac examination experience. He died of his problem about six months later prompting in me the desire for a transfer to the Chicago Navy Pier Branch of the University of Illinois, so I could be with my widowed grandmother and my mother during this trying period.

Navy Pier was approximately six miles east of my grandmother's apartment necessitating that I take a streetcar to school every day. I continued with my pre-med curriculum. Since I did not live at the school as I had at Galesburg, it was difficult to make new friends because Navy Pier was a commuter school, students arriving for their first class and leaving after their last class of the day. I would often stay after class and visit the hugh gym facility and work out or watch the gymnastic team work out; the team was the National Collegiate Athletic Association Champion featuring such famous gymnasts as Bill Rotzheim and Irving Bedard. This was a sport I knew nothing about, nor ever even witnessed before, so I became fascinated and took a gymnastics gym course. It was almost a fatal mistake. One time I tried to duplicate the gymnasts by attempting a somersault off the still rings. I landed on my head. The next thing I knew there were two gym teachers rushing toward me fully expecting to find a quadriplegic. But, I believe, God sometimes protects the ignorant and did that day. After a stern warning and a rebuke from the coaches, I stayed off the still rings. The experience made me realize that athletic skills are not God given, but come from dedication and very hard work done over a long period.

During my visits to the gym I also noted another sport that fascinated me—badminton. I need to try that, I thought. My tennis experience should come in handy. I started playing, enjoyed it very much and when they announced an intramural badminton tournament, I signed up. This sport gave me the greatest physical challenge of my life. The constant, short, explosive bursts of speed, the quick directional changes and turns were more physically exhausting than anything I had ever experienced before, and I worked my way up to the championship game. I don't want to brag, but I did make some incredible shots and won the championship which made me eligible to compete in the University of Illinois MING tournament including the champs from the Medical school, Illinois at Champaign-Urbana, Navy Pier, and Galesburg. That championship tournament did not last long for me, the winner of the Champaign-Urbana campus, my first opponent, eliminated me in the first round and went on to win the MING championship.

As it turned out, when I won the Navy Pier championship, a man I did not know who was watching the game approached me, congratulated me and asked if I ever played tennis. When I answered in the affirmative, he introduced himself as the Navy Pier tennis coach and asked me to come out for the team. This was a shock, but I answered yes and spent about a week in daily tennis practice in Grant Park until I realized that my number one priority of becoming a physician might suffer from neglecting homework. I gave my regrets to the coach, explained to him why and thus ended the chance of the United States winning the next Davis Cup.

When I completed my year at Navy Pier, I headed for Champaign-Urbana to complete my pre-med studies. The good news is that I would reestablish the relationships with my friends from Galesburg and I looked forward to that. When I was at Navy Pier, I took Algebra, did well and this made me rethink my dislike of mathematics and I decided to take more courses, meaning Analytic Geometry and Calculus. My fellow pre-meds advised against this insanity. These classes were not a pre-med requirement at the time, were difficult and not worth risking the ability to get into medical school. Not dissuaded, I viewed it as a challenge worthy of the attempt. I did very well and helped my grade point average.

The summer before I went to Champaign-Urbana, I worked for my father in his plumbing shop. My first two years, he gave me money for room, board, books and expenses. Eighty dollars per month was more than adequate to pay my twenty dollar per month room rent plus books and food, but I began to hear complaints about his ability to keep up. I told him he should stop giving me any money, because I already had a job and did not need his largesse any more. That was a blatant lie, but I was determined to get a job and make my own way. Therefore, my first order of business when I started at Champaign-Urbana was to find a job. As luck would have it, a friend of mine was a waiter and a dishwasher at a sorority house, and he got me the same position. This took care of all my food requirements; the payment was three meals per day, and since those sorority girls were well fed, so was I. It was a good job and fed me my last two years of college. Although I don't remember too much about the work details, I do remember one incident that occurred with one of the sorority girls. She was a fellow student in my analytical geometry class, but she was having her difficulties. She asked me to help her and I was pleased to do so. She sat behind me during class and I believe she looked over my shoulder when we had tests and at least once a week we got together for homework help. This went on for almost a full semester. Finally, I developed the courage to ask her for a date. Her answer, "Oh, I'm sorry, but we're not allowed to go out with the kitchen help." That certainly put me in my place.

We lived in a men's dormitory, Harmony House. This was the first year it was a men's facility. The landlady switched from a woman's home in 1949, because she tired of the "always complaining women," and believed she'd be better off with men. As it turned out, after a year of us, she switched back to women, but that's getting ahead of the story.

There was a tradition in independent men and women houses on the campus to get together on an intermittent basis for a dance, usually at the women's dorm. Someone, and I don't know who, paired up the girls and boys. This was harmless enough until one enterprising member of Harmony House set up a gambling game. Each man had to put up twenty-five cents, all the money went into a pot, the so-called "Pigpot," and the winner was the one paired up with the least physically attractive girl. My God, what hard studying students would do for entertainment! Needless to say, this created controversy, but we always solved the dilemma democratically. On one occasion, a good friend of mine returned from the date and loudly announced, "Give me the money." That evening, there was no controversy. One has to wonder if the co-eds played the same game. I hope so.

I would spend the next two years working hard to keep my grade point average within the ballpark range acceptable for a try at medical school and I succeeded while at the same time engaged in some intramural athletic activities and some innocent social life, but never with sorority girls. I had learned my lesson.

Finally, it came time to apply to medical school. A few of my friends still in pre-med applied and were accepted. I was accepted also, but as number nine alternate, which meant that if nine students of those accepted did not attend for whatever reason, but mostly because they chose another school where they were also accepted, then I would be granted admission. I waited and waited, but did not hear, so I began making arrangements to apply to graduate school in physiology where I would try for a master's degree, but never giving up on the ambition to become a physician. I had already gone back to Champaign-Urbana and purchased my graduate schoolbooks, including more math courses, when I received a call from my grandmother. She advised me that the medical school called, said I was accepted and asked if I would be able to attend. She answered, "He'll be there with bells on!" In the forty-seven years she had come from Poland with my three-month-old mother, she had learned some American colloquialism.

I sold my textbooks and vowed to remember this date as the most important day of my life, (I didn't as I think of this while writing now). I sold my textbooks, jumped into my new jalopy an old used car that burned oil excessively, purchased with the help of my uncle, Sam Siegel, that I would eventually name the Teratoma (A tumor with a variety of tissue components).

In 1951, I started medical school at the University of Illinois.

CHAPTER 8
MEDICAL SCHOOL AND INTERNSHIP

My dream fulfilled, I vowed to do my best. I followed my uncle, Sidney Tepper, who attended the University of Illinois College of Medicine and graduated in 1938. Now that I reached my first goal, I hoped to fulfill my second one—an internship at Cook County Hospital (more later).

The first year of medical school was the most important year of my life, not because of anything academic, not because of anything athletic, it had nothing to do with scholastics, nothing to do with health, nothing to do with family—but it had to do with ROMANCE. I would meet my future wife!

One evening I was studying hard when a classmate, Vernon Wallace, interrupted me suggesting that I accompany him to a dance at a nearby YMCA. "It's a nurse's dance," he advised. "But I've got all this studying to do," I replied. "Forget it," he parried, "its close and we won't stay long." This was a person who rarely took no for an answer, and I buckled under his persistence. The YMCA was located adjacent to Rush Presbyterian hospital and near Cook County hospital. We arrived...and for me things would never be the same, because simultaneously with entering the dance hall I looked to my left and saw a vision of loveliness such as I could only dream about. She was sitting on a chair against the wall with another young lady. Looking at her beautiful face struck me numb, my first thought being could I dare ask her to dance? I gathered up the courage and inquired.

"Yes," she answered. I remember very little about that dance. Subsequent discussion with her revealed that she believed I was a foreign student based upon a deep tan I had acquired during the summer at an outdoor job, and I was whistling in her ear to the dance music. She thought, what is this weirdo doing, she told me later. I learned that she was a first year nursing student from Lincoln, Nebraska at the Cook County School of Nursing across the street from the University of Illinois Medical School. Her name…Betty Lou Richards.

The location of that first meeting, the YMCA, I felt should acquire the status of a national landmark or shrine, but it wasn't to be, for within a few years the city demolished it to pave the way for the Congress Street Expressway. This crushed me, but at least the relationship lasted longer, now going on sixty-one years. Both of us would spend the next four years dating whenever we could depend upon free time in our mutual busy schedules. We married during my internship in four years (more later). I was and remain a lucky guy.

Medical school was easier and more relaxing than pre-med. I believe that had to do with the fact that the pressure to be accepted was now past history. I studied hard that first year and ended up in approximately the middle of my class causing me to relax more and study less my second year, which resulted in boosting up my standing. In those days, the first year included academic subjects such as biochemistry and gross and microscopic anatomy. The second year, along with many other courses, we started physical diagnosis and spent a full year learning how to acquire a medical history from a patient and perform a complete physical examination from "head to toe." I still feel and statistics prove that this initial physician-patient interaction will provide a diagnosis 80 percent of the time and establish a long-lasting rapport between the patient and physician. The last two years were the clinical years spending time on the various hospital and clinic services where we dealt directly with patients under the supervision of senior attending physicians.

Four years went by rapidly, I made many new friendships, most of which would end at graduation when we all went our separate ways for a year of a required internship. I never attended my own graduation because I chose an option to continue with classes during the summer semester the end of the junior year and thus was eligible to graduate three months earlier. The last year of medical school, I had my mind on one thing: acceptance at Cook County Hospital for further training—the internship—considered one of the best training hospitals in the United States and where my uncle went, although in 1938 when he graduated from medical school, two years of internship was the requirement. Since it was a city hospital, becoming an intern at Cook County required taking a competitive civil service examination. There were 120 intern slots available and 850 prospective interns took the examination, I had a one in seven chance of succeeding. How does one study for an examination of four years of medical school. You don't and just hope for the best.

This was my dream and I prayed for its fulfillment. I took the exam and waited patiently for the result. It was not long in coming. I still remember tremulously approaching the medical school bulletin board to find my standing. I ranked sixty-four out of 850—I was a Cook County Intern! Uncle Sidney, I did it. I still had a medical school graduation, but I could not attend because finishing three months early meant I had to start my internship as soon as I completed medical school. This didn't bother me because I would get my diploma anyhow, plus not going to my graduation meant that I wouldn't have to be there with my mother and father ignoring each other. This I lived to regret, because I found out many months later that my mother went to the med school graduation even though I was not there. Had I had an ounce of brains or class, I would have attended the graduation with both of my parents in attendance.

After all, it would be a fulfillment and a proud day for them, but I was too selfish. I regret it to this day, but as with any unpleasant action, I know I learned from this experience.

In those days, a rotating general internship was a requirement. You spent time in internal medicine, surgery, obstetrics and gynecology, and pediatrics along with two electives of your choice.

Dr. Karl Meyer, a general surgeon, ran the show at Cook County. He was a world famous surgeon and served as superintendent of the Cook County Hospital from 1914 to 1967, building it into a premier teaching institution sought after by interns and residents from all over the world. With 3,300 beds, usually filled, there was never a shortage of common and rare pathology of all types and rarities. I had the fortune (or misfortune) to meet Dr. Karl Meyer the first day I stepped into the hospital.

I arrived for my first day as an intern, and took an elevator to my first assignment. I got in the crowded elevator, turned to face the entrance door in front of a small man standing in the middle of the elevator, which quickly filled up with people trying to get in. The entering crowd pushed me back slamming me into the small man standing behind me who promptly slammed into the elevator back wall. I could hear the thump. The elevator went up one floor and stopped, whereupon the man who I slammed into the wall walked out staring at me the whole time. When the door closed and the elevator resumed its upward movement, a white coated person, that I presumed was a resident touched my shoulder and said, "Nice going, kid, that was Karl Meyer you just slammed against the wall." Welcome to Cook County Hospital!

The residence hall where we stayed during the year of internship, known as Karl Meyer Hall, was an excellent facility. I roomed there with a good friend and medical school classmate, Harry Dobbrunz. He already had married a nursing student and classmate of Betty's...Lily. I guess you can't get the boy out of the man because we played practical jokes on each other. One that I can remember was me taping the crotch on his undershorts making for an interesting experience when he put them on.

There were suites for two including a bathroom between both bedrooms. We ate on the main floor served cafeteria style with excellent food. In addition to this room and board, we received twenty-five dollars per month salary; the lap of luxury! Adding to that was the icing on the cake: I could look out of my bedroom window and view the Cook County School of Nursing residence...where Betty used to live! She was now an RN and gainfully employed.

I was ready to embark upon the most concentrated, intensive sleep-deprived year of my life. On the medical wards, when on call, I would "work up" as many as a dozen new patients, each one sicker than the next. On pediatrics, the same, not to mention the viral illnesses I would catch from my young patients and find myself walking back to the residence hall vomiting. On surgery I would assist on operations almost on a daily basis, and on obstetrics, I monitored daily as many as thirty women in labor and delivered over two hundred babies with all kinds of unusual presentations. It was an incredible education and experience. I quickly adjusted to the "Cook County Method of Education," watch it once, do it once, teach it."

Attending physicians, some of the most famous in Chicago, volunteered their services to make rounds with us on a regular basis, although their attendance was often spotty leaving us to fend for ourselves. There were full time chiefs of service at Cook County that we could rely on for advice; there were clinical pathological conferences held weekly where a physician assigned to discuss a case would present the history, the physical findings, laboratory and X-ray data and then, on the strength of all that clinical information, suggest the most likely diagnosis. Then the pathologist would discuss the autopsy results giving the final proven diagnosis. We would then learn if the lecturer made the diagnosis—a feather in his cap. There were also daily autopsy conferences by the department of pathology demonstrating autopsy results at 4:00 pm. These were the days when autopsies were common, the days prior to the more modern imaging and technical advances making diagnosis during life easier to establish with certainty.

This was medical education non-stop. We will never see anything like it again.

My social life was limited by the busy schedule, and on call requirements, but the good news was that Betty, who did accept a second date when we were both freshmen at our respective schools, found out that I wasn't such a creep after all. She became my steady companion. Mostly we spent time at the "Greeks," a restaurant across of the main entrance to Cook County Hospital owned by a Greek man and his three sons. It was the main hang out for the medical students, interns and residents of Cook County Hospital. We spent time in the Monkey Room where I would have a thirty-five cent beer and Betty would have a ten-cent small Van Merrit beer (sp?). You could take call at the Greeks, but the night you were on call, beer was a no-no. Occasionally, when not on call, we would jump into the Teratoma and travel to North Devon Street where Dixie Land music by the kings of this music form from around the country dazzled by their musical brilliance.

To make a long story short, I asked Betty to marry me while I was an intern (almost five years after we met at the Y). She said yes, and we married in a Synagogue on October 20th, 1955, with my father and his new wife, my mother, maternal grandmother, paternal step-grandmother, Betty's mother and assorted relatives and friend in attendance. My friend and Karl Meyer Hall room-mate, Harry Dobbrunz took movies, a prized possession to this day. My wife and I departed for a few day honeymoon at Oakton Manor across the border in Wisconsin courtesy of my father. I am indebted to Pete Pleotis, a fellow intern and medical school classmate who covered for my on call schedule, and when I asked when I could reciprocate said, "Never, it's my wedding present." Now there's a class act.

Betty and I set up housekeeping in an apartment where we paid 90 dollars per month rent, possible because of her salary of 250 dollars per month working as a visiting nurse on Skid Row. We would get ready for the next phase of our career—a two year commitment to the United States Military courtesy of a long-standing "doctor draft."

CHAPTER 9
UNITED STATES ARMY

Betty and I arrived at our first duty post for orientation. I finally had some money; the army salary was 9,000 dollars per year! We would be living high on the hog. The orientation included six weeks of medical and military education. Housing was not available on post at Fort Sam Houston Texas, so we resided in a local motel not far from the main gate. About three hundred physicians were in the class, entering as lieutenants and leaving as captains. We had lectures on military medicine, training in weaponry and military matters and went through the close combat course, crawling on our bellies while machine gun bullets fired overhead. The bullets were not my main concern, because the range master required us to walk the course first from beginning to end to "make sure there are no rattlesnakes on the course." As I crawled, with eyes fixed forward thinking of rattlesnakes, I forgot about the bullets.

In our free time, Betty and I visited the city of San Antonio, spent time in the officer's club went to movies and socialized with old and new friends. By the end of our orientation, the military authorities required that we make three choices of specialties we'd like to receive six months training in before receiving our permanent assignment. I chose my three and received radiology, which for me was an excellent choice, because I was not yet sure what specialty of medicine I wanted to devote my life to, and radiology, where you had to speak the language of all the branches of medicine, would give me a chance to make a final decision before starting a residency.

This brought Betty and I to our next assignment Fort Campbell, Kentucky, where I would receive six months of radiology training plus perform duties as a family practitioner working in radiology and the outpatient clinic. Colonel Wilson Scott, chief of radiology, proved to be an excellent teacher. Betty volunteered as a Red Cross nurse. Fort Campbell at the time was an airborne training post (101st airborne) under the command of General William Westmoreland who would go on to be the commanding general during the Viet Nam War. While posted at Fort Campbell, Betty and I would watch the paratroopers at the drop zones as they leaped out and floated to the ground. I told Betty, "Some day I'm going to do that." "Yeah, right," she replied. It took a while, but at age 75, I did a tandem jump from 14,000 feet. What a thrill!

On one occasion, we went to observe a special drop known as a heavy drop. The army set up stands around the drop zones to accommodate visiting four-star generals, the secretary of the army, Washington and local dignitaries. A heavy drop includes trucks, artillery pieces, and tanks dropped out of large planes. We watched as the massive equipment fell. They fell...and fell. When will the chutes open? I thought. They did not; the equipment, sans open chutes, hit the ground creating deep craters. I wonder whose head rolled for that mishap?

After completing my six months of radiology training, the army appointed me Chief of Radiology at Fort Sheridan, Illinois, I also had responsibility to help out in the family practice clinic after I completed my daily radiology responsibilities. Fort Sheridan, named after General Phillip Sheridan of Civil War fame, was a small military post responsible for receiving and discharging military recruits from Illinois and surrounding states. There were about 5,000 civilian and military living and working there.

Excited about returning to the Chicago area, we arrived at the Fort located in the far north suburbs of Chicago. Since there was no housing on the post, we took an apartment on the north side of Chicago and I commuted to the post every day, a half hour car ride at least. The commute occasionally became difficult, especially with traffic jams, but being back in Chicago with relatives and friends made up for it. I considered myself very lucky to be in the position I was in.

Before we arrived at Fort Sheridan and while stationed at Fort Campbell, my wife became pregnant, so we eagerly awaited the birth of our first child. She chose for her obstetrician a physician known to both of us from Cook County internship days who was now in the private practice of Obstetrics and Gynecology in Chicago. Our daughter, Gail Ellen, arrived March 10, 1957 at Augustana hospital while I bit my nails in the waiting room. My wife would have her hands full with a colicky baby, but as a mother, I could not imagine any better.

At Fort Sheridan, I was responsible for all radiology diagnostic work and if I had a problem, I could consult with the Great Lakes Naval Hospital's full time radiologist. He was most helpful. In addition, evaluating soldiers and their dependents in the family practice clinic kept me abreast of patient diagnosis and treatment.

CHAPTER 10
RESIDENCY

I completed my tour of duty at Fort Sheridan, and while there decided that I would start a radiology residency at Cook County Hospital, my previous internship there guaranteeing my acceptance. The disadvantage was the fact that I reverted to pauperhood, my salary dropping from 9,000 dollars per year to 125 dollars per month, not enough to support a wife and child. Betty wanted to go to work, but I think we both agreed that a colicky baby was enough of a full time job. I would find a job and work my evenings off as much as possible. The 'as much as possible' plus the residency requirements plus private practice for many years would prompt my wife to respond to the question years later, "What kept you guys together so long?" with the answer, "That was easy, I never saw him for forty years."

I came into a radiology residency much better pre-pared than the average starting radiology resident. After all, I entered the program with almost two years of expe-rience in the military. I even brought copies of very un-usual X-ray films. The radiology department's chief was happy to have me join the program, so I found it a bit difficult to tell him after three months that I wanted to switch residencies to Internal Medicine for I missed the direct patient contact, the histories and physicals, the attempt at diagnosis. The chief of medicine welcomed me and said I would receive internal medicine credit for my three months of radiology, but I had to spend the first three months on a geriatric service at a County hospital situated on the far south side. This meant a forty-five minute commute both ways, and staying there when on call. But the time went fast, and I returned to Cook County Hospital to start the usual medical rotations. This plus the inner city clinic evening work I found allowed me to eke out a living and pay my bills. Continuing to live on the north side of Chicago and with my family nearby, Betty and I could rely on occasional social, some financial and baby-sitting support.

The hospital had not changed much in the intervening three years. The voluminous medical diagnostic puzzles kept flooding in straining our brains on a daily basis, but that is what it's all about and that was what I had missed the most. When my wife told her obstetrician that Sheldon had switched from radiology to medicine, his only comment was "Well, that just cost him 100,000 dollars per year." During the residency, Betty gave birth to our son, Paul, on September 19, 1959, at Illinois Masonic Hospital, delivered by the same obstetrician. Now we had two blessed children.

When one is as busy as Betty and I were, time passes before your eyes, the residency was over, the year was 1961, and we had to make a decision about private practice. Also one more hurdle to surmount was the need to take internal medicine boards two years after being in private practice and consisting of two parts: written one year and if passed, an oral examination the next year consisting in the evaluation of two patients.

CHAPTER 11
PRIVATE PRACTICE

The first order of business was to make it possible to find a home where we could raise a growing family. On the strength of a 3,000 dollar down-payment loan from my mother, we purchased a house in Morton Grove, Illinois, a northwest suburb of Chicago. The second order of business would be to establish a private practice. Two friends, also completing an internal medicine residency had the same thought and we all made what would prove to be a mistake; we rented office space in Park Ridge, Illinois with the idea of sharing expenses, on call time, and building up individual practices. We all worked in inner city clinics and now that the residency was completed, we could work more time enabling an increased income to support us while we "built up the practices." This was naiveté to the extreme. To make a long story short—it did not work. One of my "associates," while an internal medicine resident, made over a million dollars during his residency mastering the stock market. Need I say where his focus of attention was? He became a full time investor and part time physician. The other associate was in the same shoes as mine. He worked at an inner-city clinic, purchased a home in the suburbs, raised a family and, like me, spent much time in his car. Rookie mistakes. The icing on the cake for me was an interesting episode that taught me a valuable lesson. Making hospital rounds on one patient, I started a paroxysm of coughing. I did not feel well for several days, but had to keep working. The patient said, and I quote, "Boy, you look like s—t, better go down and take an X-ray." I did. The diagnosis: pneumonia. A colleague hospitalized me, started me on antibiotics and confirmed that I had a severe mycoplasma pneumonia diagnosed by a massive elevation of my cold-agglutinin titer of 4,096, the highest I had ever seen. I dragged for about six weeks and made a full recovery, but also made a decision to stop my traveling, vagabond existence and settle into a single practice along with one other intellectually stimulating exercise: I was also an attending physician at Cook County Hospital. Now it was my turn to teach residents and interns on a part time, unsalaried basis.

The prevailing private practice fees those days were five dollars an office visit, five dollars per hospital visit, the government paid two dollars per visit for public aid patients and when Medicare started, the office visit fee was three dollars. How times have changed!

As it so happened, I had a friend, an obstetrician who had an office building in Addison, Illinois, and was after me to rent space in his building suggesting that the community needed an internist. I took him up on the offer, left the Park Ridge office, and discovered that my friend was correct. My newly established practice flourished. Now I had an office and a part time teaching assignment. One difficulty remained: the extremely overcrowded hospital close to the Addison community had a closed medical staff and a moratorium on new doctors. This meant that I would still have a long commute to distant hospitals. The good news was that a new and close hospital on the drawing board would allow me to have an office and hospital in close proximity to each other. I could look forward to better days ahead, anxiously awaiting the arrival of the Alexian Brothers Elk Grove village hospital close to my Addison office.

After two years in practice, I was eligible to take the American Board of Internal Medicine written test. I studied the entire Cecil's textbook of medicine and the latest internal medicine literature. I passed. One year later, they scheduled me to take the oral examinations at Cook County Hospital. Two internists quizzed me individually, each with a different patient. The second patient was very complicated, and had extensive X-ray evaluation and multiple diagnoses. After discussing the diagnoses in detail, I sensed the examiner was satisfied and we had time, so he thumbed through the X-ray reports on the charts and pulled the X-Rays out of the X-ray file box, gave them to me while he held the written paper report and asked me to, " read that X-ray and tell me what it shows."

I was in seventh heaven and as I described the X-ray films, I could see his facial expression: one of amazement that I knew so much. He kept giving me film after film for twenty minutes. When finished, he said, "I never knew any internist who was so superb in X-ray interpretation. I thanked him electing not to mention my two years of X-ray training ;-). There was no way I was going to flunk.

The Alexian Brothers are a Catholic order started in the Middle Ages in Europe consisting of men and women who banded together to tend to the sick, help the poor and unfortunate, and bury the dead during plagues. By 1472, Pope Sixtus V confirmed the Alexian Brothers as a religious community. In the last 600 years, they spread their mission all over the world including the United States with the arrival of Brother Bonaventure Thelen in Chicago, Illinois, in 1866. He established a small hospital, and from there, after its destruction in the Chicago fire, the Alexian Brothers built a large fire-proof hospital on Belden Avenue, Chicago. In the early 1960's, they moved to Elk Grove Village and today, as of this writing in 2012, they have a comprehensive health network consisting of Alexian Brother's Medical Center in Elk Grove Village, Alexian Brother's Rehabilitation Hospital in Elk Grove Village, St. Alexius Medical Center in Hoffman Estates, Alexian Brother's Behavioral Health Hospital in Hoffman Estates, and Alexian Brother's center for Mental Health in Arlington Heights.

In preparation for the as yet not built hospital, I joined their Chicago hospital staff, waited for them to close and this automatically made me a staff member of Alexian Brother's hospital in Elk Grove Village. I was ready to admit patients. One might say I christened the hospital; I admitted the first patient—and this is a story in itself.

The first day the hospital was ready to receive in-patients, I was in my office that early morning when a walk-in patient arrived, reported she was ill and asked to "see the doctor." She was a very attractive twenty-three-year-old circus acrobat from out of town. Her chief complaints were cough and chills. I took a history and did a physical examination and the main findings were temperature of 102 and rales (crackling sounds) in the right lung base consistent with the diagnosis of pneumonia. I called up the admitting office of the new hospital and admitted her—patient number one. I wrote orders and told her I would see her later. The X-ray did confirm the pneumonia and after testing, including a blood culture, I started her on intravenous penicillin. When I saw her that afternoon, she was resting comfortably and had the entire floor to herself for a time. The next morning, her temperature was 100 and she stated she felt better. The third day, I received a call from an assistant administrator advising me that I needed to, "Please discharge the patient." This was a first; never had anyone from any hospital hierarchy call and advise a discharge, purely a medical decision. I responded, "She's improving for sure, but not yet ready for discharge. I'd like to be certain her temperature completely resolves. Perhaps in a day or two? Why do you want me to discharge her please?" I asked. "Because the nurse caught her in bed with the married man in the next room."

The two patients, probably the only ones on the floor that first day, found each other. I have to wonder if that man, whoever he was, bragged about the service.

From these 'humble' beginnings, the hospital would evolve into a major healthcare network in about forty years while at the same time expanded their world-wide ministry

Now I had the best of all worlds; one hospital, one office, one solo practice, hopefully no more pneumonias, and more than enough to do for a primary care general internist. The practice grew at a steady pace. I became the leading internal medicine consultant, at least until the subspecialties of internal medicine evolved over the years. In addition, I took in my first physician associate. Now I would not have to take call twenty-four hours per day, 7 days per week.

In the early seventies, the expanding hospital announced the construction of a large physician office building extending from the main hospital. I was the first one to sign up for a suite. The thought of one location for every aspect of your office and hospital practice was too attractive to ignore. My associate and I moved in and in time, two more internists joined us. The office, of course was much larger and the necessity to care for an emergency hospital patient was now just a short walk 'down the hall,' an extremely efficient way to practice medicine assuring the quickest response possible to meet urgent patient demand.

While my mind wrapped up in medicine as it was, I can only thank God that I had a wife who put her career on hold and paid attention to family and children. Whatever success our children acquired is due to her efforts. When they grew up, she went back to school to continue her nursing education, acquire a bachelor's degree and master's degree, made the nursing honor society and worked as director of nursing education at a Chicago hospital.

Direct patient care was not the only things physicians and hospitals needed to be concerned about. After

World War II and into the sixty's, medical care changes, medical care economics, government responsibility, physician responsibility, medico-legal issues, financial issues were all coalescing to force major changes on hospitals and physicians. The future of health delivery was at stake.

CHAPTER 12
MEDICAL CARE DELIVERY

All hospitals have governing bodies. In years back, Hospital Board of Trustees assumed responsibility for hospital operation and left the quality of medical care in the institution to the doctors. After all, what did lay trustees know about the care of patients? The doctors grew up in this milieu, giving this over-all responsibility little thought while involved in one on one patient decision-making on an hourly basis. Their mind set was to leave the running of the hospital physical plant, employees, finances to trustees, a doctor's job is to care for patients and the less interference with this sacred task, the better. This was the established system until pressure appeared from multiple sources forcing rethinking of this mode of operation. What were these pressures?

The first example I will give is a legal case known as Darling v. Charleston Community Hospital. On November 6, 1960, an eighteen year old broke his leg playing college football. Brought to the emergency room, an on-call physician, with the assistance of hospital personnel, applied traction and placed the leg in a plaster cast with a heat cradle to dry the cast. Subsequently the patient experienced great pain and his toes became swollen, turned dark and eventually cold and insensitive. That evening the doctor "notched' the cast around the toes, and the following day, the doctor cut the cast three inches up from the foot. On November 8, he split the sides of the cast with a Stryker saw, and unfortunately cut the patient's leg. The nurses observed blood and other seepage plus a stench emanating from the leg. They patient remained in the hospital for about a week and then his physician transferred him to Barnes hospital in St Louis. Several surgeries performed in an attempt to save the leg were unsuccessful, necessitating an 8 inch below the knee amputation.

The plaintiff attorney contended: the hospital was negligent in permitting the doctor to do orthopedic work; the doctor was negligent in his therapy and failure to call consultation; the nurses were negligent in not watching the patient's toes for color and temperature changes; the hospital administration was negligent for not supervising nurses, not bringing the problem to the attention of the medical staff, and not following their own bylaws.

The defendant's position was that "It is a fundamental rule of law that only an individual properly educated and licensed, and not a corporation, may practice medicine. Accordingly, a hospital is powerless under the law to forbid or command any act by a physician or surgeon in the practice of his profession. A hospital is not an insurer of their patient's recovery, but only owes the patient the duty to exercise such reasonable care as his known condition requires and that degree of care, skill and diligence used by hospitals in that community. Where the evidence shows that the hospital care was in accordance with standard practice obtaining in similar hospitals, and plaintiff produces no evidence to the contrary, the jury cannot conclude that the opposite is true even if they disbelieve the hospital witnesses. A hospital is not liable for the torts of its nurse committed while the nurse was but executing the orders of the patient's physician, unless such order is so obviously negligent as to lead any reasonable person to anticipate that substantial injury would result to the patient from the execution of such order. The extent of the duty of a hospital with respect to actual medical care of a professional nature such as is furnished by a physician is to use reasonable care in selecting medical doctors. When such care in the selection of the staff is accomplished, and nothing indicates that a physician so selected is incompetent or that such incompetence should have been discovered, more cannot be expected from the hospital administration.

A few hospital boards became sensitive to these unexpected and unwelcome responsibilities. Alexian Brothers was the leader amongst them. Most physicians saw this as a threat to their authority and started to dig in their heels. If that wasn't enough, there were other pressures on doctor and hospitals, causing them to rethink the entire topic of responsibility for medical care. They are:

- The cost of medical care rose at an unprecedented rate between 1960 and 1970, increasing faster than any other part of the Consumer Price Index. In 1950, the cost of medical care for the year was $12 billion. In 1970, over $72 billion. Big money in those days; sounds like loose change today in 2012.

- State, federal government, labor unions, insurance companies, third party payers, individuals became increasingly concerned about better care, less costly care, and easier access to care. Congress became concerned. The House Ways and Means Committee held hearings.

- Demand for better control of the healthcare system.

- Demand for new and less costly modes of delivery—Health Maintenance Organizations

- Demands for improvements in the present mode of medical delivery

All these ingredients including the Darling case made for a health care crisis that cried out for solution

Before the Alexian Brothers built their new hospital in Elk Grove Village in 1966, they approached local practicing physicians from the closest hospital. They sought their assistance developing medical staff bylaws. This assistance, of course, came from many long-standing practicing physicians steeped in the philosophy of physician control of hospitals. A hospital was a "physician's workshop" where physicians practiced medicine as they pleased unencumbered by any authority. This group of physicians, working with the brothers, established medical staff bylaws that reflected this mindset—and those were the medical staff bylaws with which the hospital, known as St. Alexius hospital at the time, started to function.

I was not part of that original medical staff bylaw group, and I was already a staff member entering through the back door based upon my membership on the staff of the original Chicago Alexian Brother's hospital. Since I became one of the largest admitter of patients and this was the only hospital I used, I had a vested interest in its quality. I was very sympathetic to the doctrine of Board of Trustee authority including responsibility for medical care, but most of the older physicians viewed it as a threat.

Physicians took sides, the vast majority preferring to keep the existing system. I firmly believed that changes were coming and it made sense that a board of a hospital corporation needed to assume responsibility for all phases of its operation. Granted, the lay board members could not practice medicine, but they had the responsibility to assure that they put mechanisms in place that would guarantee to the greatest extent possible that all physicians practiced quality medical care. With professional consultants called in, with group meetings organized, the consensus was that the loose medical staff organization, the very busy physicians, many of them going to 2 or 3 hospitals could not possibly have the time to assume full responsibility for as important an undertaking as hospital based quality care.

To this point, physician officers of the staff were elected by physicians; the president of the staff for a one year term of office elected at one of the quarterly staff meetings; department chairmen elected for a one year term at one of the departmental meetings. This system was a non-system. It was unsalaried, it was voluntary, and no busy physician, especially those on multiple hospital staffs, had the time to pay attention to details. Whoops, there's a problem? Well, I'm almost finished with my term of office. I'll let the next guy take care of it. With all the changes and demands on healthcare, that was no longer tenable. The concept of board of trustee authority for running all aspects of their hospital including assuring medical care quality was a no-brainer to me, and I emerged as the leader of this movement. Enemies surfaced. My wife received a phone call at home advising that, "If your husband didn't cease and desist his activities, he will…she hung up.

After many meetings including medical staff organizational seminars in and out of town, consultants, medical bylaw drafting committee meetings, a new set of medical staff bylaws and hospital bylaws, set the stage for a reorganization where all divisions of a hospital including physicians, nursing, ancillary personnel, hospital management, financial, would work together for the collaborative good to put quality measures in place assuring a smooth functioning system geared to quality medical care. The efforts received national publicity appearing in magazines and newspapers. The Board of Trustees realized that part-time non-salaried doctors could not be responsible for such organization, so part and full time salaried doctors, appointed by the Board of Trustees with physician input would now be responsible for medical staff quality and work together with the hospital for performance improvement activities.

Due to my leadership work on these committees, the board of Trustees appointed me medical director. Many older physicians, inactive for the most part, resigned. It took about two years to lower the decibel level, and after four years, I resigned to be able to continue full time practice. I would return as medical director in about eleven years for a period of five years. Then, at the age of sixty-five, I retired from the active practice of medicine. As of this writing, our children are in their fifties, my daughter a speech pathologist, my son an attorney and CPA with an LLM in tax, six grandchildren, and two great grandchildren.

I would not trade my life and the practice of medicine for anything! I'll give you an idea why in the next chapter where I tell about some unusual medical cases.

CHAPTER 13
CASE REPORTS

These are cases that I remember from my years as a medical student, intern, resident and private practitioner. They also include some cases told to me by colleagues. I hope it illustrates the variety of patients that the average primary care physician will experience over time. If you are a young reader thinking about a medical career, I hope it will influence you to become a physician, or other member of the healthcare team.

I have already published these patient case reports in an electronic book as examples of how a careful medical history and physical examination can of itself lead to a diagnosis—The Slim Book of Health Pearls: THE COMPLETE MEDICAL EXAMINATION (cohenebooks.com). Sir William Osler, the most famous pioneering internist of all time said, "Let the patient talk, doctor, she's trying to give you the diagnosis." The cases follow and reflect diagnoses made from aspects of the medical history and the physical examination.

A teenaged boy developed abdominal pain associated with an elevated temperature. The pain started in the right lower part of his belly and then spread throughout his entire abdomen. Hospitalized with the presumptive diagnosis of appendicitis, his symptoms resolved before contemplated surgery and his physician discharged him. He had another similar attack four months later, which again resolved, and based upon the region of the world his mother and father came from—North Africa—his physician made a final diagnosis, a genetic illness, familial Mediterranean fever, caused by a defect on a specific gene and occurs in North African Arabs, Sephardic Jews, Armenians, Turks, Greeks and Italians. There is therapy that provides excellent improvement in symptoms and marked reduction in the complication rate.

This is an example of how the biographical data including the origin and ethnicity led to the proper diagnosis.

A young African-American man developed severe pain in his lower legs, his lumbar spine and his abdomen, raising suspicion of sickle cell anemia. This condition was not a rare event at Cook County Hospital where I trained, and occurs in African Americans for the most part. The characteristic findings on his complete blood count led to the diagnosis. Sickle cell anemia is a hereditary condition where red blood cells, instead of being the normal round shape, are sickle shaped. These abnormal cells can clog blood capillaries causing a variety of symptoms including pain. Proper therapy has prolonged life in these patients.

It was the patient's race, in this instance, that led to a diagnosis.

Sometimes the first sentence of the medical history is enough to make a diagnosis. "I feel weak, I lost ten pounds, and I'm thirsty all the time." A quick urinalysis followed by a blood sugar test confirmed the diagnosis of diabetes mellitus. In this instance, the three facts of the chief complaint led to a presumptive diagnosis proven by the follow-up tests.

"It feels like an elephant stepped on my chest." The patient had what sounded like angina—chest pain due to a blocked coronary artery or arteries. Coronary artery angiography (X-ray of coronary arteries using opaque dye) was confirmatory. His anterior descending coronary artery was almost completely blocked. He underwent successful cardiac surgery. The patient's classical description of angina pectoris confirmed the diagnosis with a high degree of certainty. Other diagnoses may be responsible for such a description by the patient, but the first and most important cause may be cardiac in origin and ruled out as soon as possible.

Many years ago as an intern at Cook County Hospital's Fantus Clinic, on a follow up visit, a patient's chief complaint was, "I'm not any better. I couldn't take the stuff you prescribed." "Why?" I asked. "Well, I managed to swallow those big pills, but trying to get that liquid down was impossible—yuck." This was not exactly the route I had in mind when I prescribed vaginal suppositories and a vaginal douche.

The patient's chief complaint was "bad headache." Details of the present illness revealed that these headaches awakened the patient in the middle of the night. The pain was severe, one-sided and described as being "around the right eye and in front of and above the ear." It lasted about an hour. Also associated with the pain was a flood of tears from the effected eye. These medical history details were enough to make the diagnosis of cluster headaches, an illness of unknown etiology, but amenable to acute and long-term preventive therapy.

Here again is another example of the patient's chief complaint yielding a prompt and correct diagnosis. The patient's chief complaint was "having trouble hearing." The details of the present illness revealed that the patient was experiencing some hearing deficits when she found that she had to turn her head to understand what people were saying. The onset of this symptom seemed to be rather abrupt. This abruptness prompted further questions, and it was determined that she also noted persistent ringing in the involved ear, a feeling of fullness, some loss of equilibrium and headache. All these details were suspicious for the diagnosis of acoustic neuroma, a tumor of the eighth cranial, or acoustic nerve, the nerve responsible for hearing. This diagnosis, suspected by the details of the history, would not have been possible without asking the proper questions. The patient's answers led to a prompt search for the tumor. Studies verified the tumor. A neurosurgeon successfully removed it.

On the other hand, here is what could happen when you don't take a careful present illness. As a young intern, I was working a twelve-hour shift in Chicago's Cook County Hospital's emergency department. This was a solid twelve hours of work, as I never remember the waiting room emptying out. A middle-aged man's chief complaint was that he was "Having trouble with my nose."

We spent much of our time in this busy location taking direct care of patients and triaging many patients to the proper medical clinic. In this case, during a very busy time, I told the patient with the "nose trouble" that we would send him to the Ear Nose and Throat clinic for care. About an hour passed and the ENT resident came down to the emergency room and told me to come to the ENT clinic so I could see the man I sent to him with the "nose trouble." His serious demeanor prompted a quick acquiescence on my part. My God, I thought, what did I miss? When we arrived, I saw the patient, stooped over with his hands on his lap seated on the examining table. The resident spoke to the patient and said, "Tell this doctor about your nose, sir." The patient responded, "Well you see, doc, my nose keeps getting longer and longer until it gets all the way out here." The patient extended his right arm full length forward. "And then it gets so heavy I fall over."

That story just did not stop there. My good friend—the ENT resident—spread it around the hospital. All I could hope is that others, as well as myself, learned the importance of acquiring a thorough present illness as part of the medical history. Yes, the patient at last got the right referral—to the neuro-psychiatric department.

In the early days of the discovery of HIV, when physicians only made the diagnosis on homosexuals, a man came into my office complaining of a sore mouth. It was clear he had thrush, a yeast infection caused by candida albicans. I asked him about his sexual preference. He told me he was homosexual. His HIV test was positive. Since these early days, HIV has become an international health problem affecting anyone regardless of sexual preference.

Paramedics transported an unconscious young man to the emergency room. He was in status epilepticus, a state of persistent, unrelenting convulsive seizures. Specific therapy over an extended time resolved his seizures. When he regained consciousness, he had no idea how he got to the hospital, nor what had happened to him. He denied ever having had a seizure before. The initial impression in a young man with sudden onset of a first seizure would be a brain tumor, but further questioning failed to reveal any other symptoms suggestive of this diagnosis. Nevertheless, that did not rule it out, and tests done to determine if this was the diagnosis were negative. He had no recollection of his pre-seizure activities. A day went by and his memory returned, and when questioned again about immediate pre-seizure recollections, his eyes opened wide. "Oh God, I remember," he said. "I took cocaine for the first time." That made the diagnosis. I asked him if he was a religious man. "Not really," he answered. I suggested, however, that he should go to the church of his choice and thank God that he was alive. Any repetition of the same behavior, based upon what happened his first time, could mean he might be performing the last act of his life. He was very grateful—and one could only pray he learned his lesson.

A pale, short teenager complained of fatigue and easy bruising. A blood count confirmed that the patient was anemic. He also had a low platelet count, which explained his easy bruising tendency. In this age group, one would have to be concerned about leukemia or other blood disease, but the fact that the patient was Jewish, and his grandparents came from Eastern Europe, meaning that he was an Ashkenazi Jew, suggested the diagnosis of Gaucher's disease. This is an inherited metabolic disorder where certain fatty substances accumulate in the liver, spleen and bone marrow. Gaucher's disease was confirmed. There is effective enzyme therapy to control this genetic error. The family history was the clue to the diagnosis.

A senior citizen came to the office complaining of left arm pain. He had the pain, on occasion, after he injured the nerve under his left arm while sprinting around a corner when jogging about five years ago. He felt a "rip in my left arm pit." The next two days he had a left hand weakness, diagnosed as a left brachial plexus nerve injury. From that time on, he experienced occasional left arm pain, which eventually became more frequent. Left arm pain can be indicative of angina, but the patient had no other cardiac symptoms. He attributed the arm pain to a "flare up of the nerve injury." However, his family history did reveal his maternal grandfather to have died of "heart block." Further questioning also revealed that his grandfather's four brothers "all died of heart attacks in their sixties." The patient failed a cardiac stress test ordered on the strength of this important family history data. A coronary artery angiogram demonstrated a major narrowing of his left anterior descending branch of the left coronary artery plus some lesser blocks involving other coronary arteries. He underwent multiple coronary bypass grafts, made an uneventful recovery and is doing well. The family history, in this case, was the clue to turn attention away from a brachial plexus injury and toward a cardiac origin.

A forty six year old woman complained of constant fatigue. "Sometimes I have to park in a parking lot and go to sleep for a half hour. When I wake up in the morning I feel like I should be going to bed now." Detailed questioning about her sleep habits prompted the ordering of a sleep study, which confirmed the diagnosis of obstructive sleep apnea. She could not tolerate the sleep masks used as treatment, and a dental appliance did not work. On her own she discovered a sensitivity to gluten, a protein found in wheat and other grains, and since she went gluten-free, her sleep apnea improved and a follow-up X-ray of her throat revealed a wider air passage. My inquiry of sleep specialists revealed that they had not heard of this possible etiology of sleep apnea, but the patient insists on her improvement since going gluten-free.

An executive of a large company underwent a corporate physical examination. His blood profile demonstrated an abnormal elevation of three liver enzymes. He came to me in consultation as to the significance of these abnormalities. He stated he was a married man with children and had never received a blood transfusion or had taken illegal drugs. He had a negative history, but the abnormal enzymes prompted questions of alcohol intake. He said he only drank at lunch. "How much?" I asked. "Two a day and none on weekends when I'm home, unless I go out to dinner, then I might have one or two." "What do you drink?" I asked. "Martinis," he replied. I told him that physicians have learned to double or triple what a patient tells them if they want to come up with the right amount. He persisted and swore that he never had more than two a day. He would not change his story. I examined him and told him that he did indeed have an enlarged liver. "What does that mean?" he asked. "It could be a fatty liver resulting from early alcohol liver damage, or cirrhosis from alcohol, or even other liver problems such as hepatitis, but I have to confess it would be unusual for two drinks a day to cause alcohol liver disease." "How could I find out if alcohol has anything to do with it?" he asked. I told him my recommendation would be to stop drinking 100%, and repeat the tests in two months. If it was from the alcohol, the tests should return to normal by then. "Is there a faster way?" he asked. "Yes, a liver biopsy, but I wouldn't recommend it." "Why not?" "Because the procedure is not risk free." "What could happen?" "You could bleed from it, and sometimes that bleeding is life threatening, so the test is not done unless the information is a must." "I want to have it done," he said. To make a long story short—he insisted, so I referred him to a gastroenterologist and waited to see if the gastroenterologist would agree to perform the biopsy. He did, and the biopsy was positive for alcoholic cirrhosis, a chronic condition and called into question his "two drinks a day." Since I only saw him in consultation, the patient took his records and went back to his regular physician in an adjacent town. I hope he learned from it and stopped alcohol.

A concerned mother brought her high school student son to my office. He had lost ten pounds, and, "Lost all his ambition." I took the young man's history, did a complete physical and found nothing wrong. I told his mother this, and then said I would order tests to be sure of my impression. As the young man looked depressed, I asked his mother if I could speak with her son alone for a while. She agreed. As it turned out, he was distraught over the loss of a girlfriend that "dumped me for another guy." It reminded me of patients I had taken care of who had gone through a bitter divorce. Since I had been "dumped" by perhaps one young woman in my youth, I could relate and be a good counselor. With talk sessions, and an exercise program, the young man resolved the issue, regained his weight and did not require antide-pressants.

A middle-aged woman developed a chronic and severe cough. It interfered with her work. She is a speech pathologist and visits clients in their homes. She also had a part time job working in a grade school. The cough was so severe her family physician referred her to a pulmonologist (lung specialist) who diagnosed asthma, or to be more specific—cough variant asthma, and loaded her up with medications and an inhaler. She spoke to me about it, not as a patient but as a friend, and my only comment was that I could not dispute the pulmonologist's diagnosis, but I did not like the new wording for what physicians, in prior times, called allergic bronchitis. I felt that the asthma title labeled the patient as chronic, and could prevent future health insurance. I did, however, tell her that her mother, who was a brilliant former nurse, had a point when she suggested a diagnosis. The patient's mother had made her own medical observation based upon the patient's social history: "When did the coughing start," the mother asked. "About a year ago," was the patient's answer. "Wasn't that about when you started working at the school?" "Yes, do you think that has something to do with it?" the patient asked. "Maybe. Don't you work in one room where you see the kids who come to you for speech problems?" "Yes, I do." "I bet you're allergic to something in that room," the mother said. This was about the time when the patient found it necessary to quit the part-time school job—and sure enough, the cough resolved. The summer passed and the patient visited the schoolroom where she had seen the children, and she found the walls torn down in that entire wing of the school. She started coughing for the first time in three months, and asked a friend, "What happened here?" "Oh, they had to tear the whole place down," she replied. "How come?" "They found black mold in the walls." There was the answer to the patient's former problem, which resolved when she left the exposure to the mold. This case also illustrates the fact that a nurse can take an excellent history and a physician can miss important facts! This is a perfect example of why patients must take charge of their health and always seek answers—and with the coming healthcare changes, now more than ever. (See my new book The Coming Healthcare Revolution: Take Control of Your Health).

Four members of an African American family visited the dermatology clinic at Cook County Hospital—a man, his wife, and two teen aged children. The husband of the patient stated that he brought his wife because "her skin was getting darker and darker." Indeed, the patient's husband and the two children had relatively light skin. The wife and mother appeared almost "pitch black." The patient also complained of severe fatigue, and her blood pressure was 90/56. These symptoms plus evidence of low adrenal hormone production via blood test confirmed the diagnosis of Addison's disease, or adrenal gland under activity (an autoimmune disease). The patient received cortisone replacement therapy to supply the hormone that her own adrenal glands could no longer make.

A middle-aged man presented with a single symptom of diffuse itching. A complete medical history and physical examination was unremarkable except for some signs of skin irritation induced by the patient's intense scratching. The symptoms would remit and exacerbate. After about a year, he developed a neck mass, biopsy of which was determined to be Hodgkin's disease. This is a lymph gland malignancy with a good prognosis if caught early. With therapy for his underlying disease the patient's itching stopped. In this case, the cause of the itching could not be determined until the patient had developed enlarged lymph nodes.

A female graduate student complained of sudden onset of bilateral milk-like nipple discharge. She was unmarried and had not missed any menstrual periods. Bilateral nipple discharge is due to increased prolactin hormone production from the pituitary gland. She had no other symptoms. She often "smoked a joint" with some friends. She went on the internet, did a Google search and discovered that galactorrhea is the medical term for bilateral nipple discharge. She did another Google search for galactorrhea, and found a list of the causes— one of which was marijuana. She stopped the marijuana, and the nipple discharge disappeared. In this case, she took charge of her health and was her own advocate.

A middle-aged woman complained of a one-month history of a rust-colored nipple discharge from the right breast. Physical examination revealed only some mild tenderness, but no palpable mass. A mammogram was negative, but the possibility of the patient having an early malignancy was good since the discharge was coming from one duct. A surgeon operated. She had a carcinoma-in-situ, which is a very early cancer involving only the cell lining of the duct. Her prognosis is excellent.

A senior citizen male came to the office complaining, "I got blind in one eye. It was like a curtain came over it. It only lasted about a minute." This is a classical description of amaurosis fugax—amaurosis from the Greek meaning dark, and fugax from the Latin meaning fleeting. This symptom suggests a vascular cause, but there are other causes, including eye diseases, migraine and other illnesses. The main cause is a stroke until proven otherwise and this should prompt an evaluation of the blood vessels to the brain. In this patient's case, there were no major blood vessel blockages, there were no abnormalities on the neurological or eye examination, and there was no history of migraine. The presumptive diagnosis was a transient ischemic cerebral attack, meaning a temporary blockage of an artery to the brain due to spasm or clot.

A woman came to the office with multiple complaints, one of which was eye pain. She underwent a complete examination including a cursory eye exam. One of the more common causes of eye pain is glaucoma. If untreated, it can lead to blindness. In glaucoma, the interior eye fluid is under increased pressure. The measurement of this pressure requires an instrument that is often not available in a primary care physician's office. A rough estimate of the pressure is possible by having the patient close her eyes. The doctor then touches the closed eyelids with the tip of the second and middle finger and gently presses on the eyeball. In the normal patient, the eyeballs are soft and give a little under the pressing finger. With glaucoma, the increased pressure causes the eyeballs to be more rigid and this was my impression. That is only presumptive evidence, however, but the ophthalmologist confirmed the presence of glaucoma. In the majority of cases, treatment is very effective.

A middle-aged Chinese man came to the office with complaints of increasing right-sided nasal blockage and occasional bloody nasal drainage. Examination revealed two hard and firm lymph glands on both sides of the upper neck. An examination of his exterior nasal passages was unrevealing. A referral to an ear, nose, and throat specialist confirmed the diagnosis of nasopharyngeal carcinoma, not an uncommon malignancy in people of Chinese ancestry.

A patient came to my office for a complete medical examination. The chief complaint was gastrointestinal in nature. In taking a system review, the patient stated that he had nasal congestion for years, but "I live with it." Examination of his nose revealed polyps appearing like many 'seedless grapes' obstructing his nasal passageway—an allergic condition. An ear, nose and throat specialist removed the polyps offering the patient considerable relief. This case demonstrates that a well-taken system review (evaluation of each organ system by medical history) can elicit problems not related to the patient's chief complaint.

A middle-aged woman came to the office with a chief complaint of fatigue and joint pains. The system review did elicit the fact that her "mouth was always dry and I carry a water bottle with me wherever I go." Based on the symptoms described, I made a diagnosis of Sjogren's syndrome. This is an autoimmune inflammatory disorder characterized by dry mouth, dry eyes, arthritis, plus a long list of other possible symptoms. The disease is chronic and incurable, but the symptoms are treatable. The patient was at least relieved to discover that she "wasn't a neurotic after all."

A young man came to the emergency room of Cook County hospital in severe distress complaining of a sore throat. He was holding his neck and jaw with his left hand. He was grimacing exemplifying the agony he was experiencing. When asked what was wrong, he could only point to his throat. He had difficulty opening his mouth, but I did manage to get an adequate look and discovered a large left-sided peritonsillar abscess. The normal anatomy, distorted by this large pus-filled mass almost extended to the other side obstructing his throat. This is a severe, but rare complication of a sore throat gone unattended. However, there is nothing as gratifying to the patient and the doctor as to see the immediate relief that ensues when the pus spouts out of the incised abscess and a smile comes over the relieved patient's face.

An elderly female complained of fatigue and bilateral knee pain limiting her ability to walk. In taking the medical history, it was apparent that her voice was very hoarse. "Oh, no, I always talk that way," she said. "Do you smoke?" "Yes, she responded. Both she and her husband had smoked for sixty years. I asked her husband and daughter if they did not think the patient's voice was hoarse. They assured me that "that's the way she's always talked," and seemed a little irritated that I was zeroing in on an unimportant issue not related to the purpose of her visit. Seeing their response, I concentrated on the patient's chief complaints. When they left, I did recommend that they see an ear nose and throat specialist just to be sure there was no problem with her vocal cords, because there was always a possibility that loved ones who hear her talking every day could miss a very slow evolving hoarseness. They did see the specialist who found several polyps on her vocal cords requiring surgical removal. They were benign. Neither she nor her husband has stopped smoking. This is another example of where a symptom not related to the patient's chief complaint resulted in important information.

A college student came to the office complaining of severe sore throat, fever and fatigue. In looking in his throat, there were petechiae at the junction of his hard and soft palate. These tiny red blood spots, caused by minute hemorrhages, when taken together with a severe sore throat are classical for infectious mononucleosis. Blood tests confirmed the diagnosis. This is a viral disease and time and rest are curative.

When I was in medical school, one of my professors told us about a patient whom he saw in consultation. This middle-aged man was in chronic heart failure. In those days, all that was available for heart failure was a toxic mercury-based diuretic known as mercuhydrin, digitalis and a low salt diet. Cardiac surgery was not yet available. The long-term prognosis for patients with this diagnosis was poor—their life expectancy was about two years. Nowadays, of course, there is very effective life prolonging therapy. After the patient was seen, and my professor made what recommendations he could, the patient thanked him and said, "Well, now back to the salt mines." The professor chuckled, thinking he meant he was going back to work, but he asked the patient, "Oh, what kind of work do you do now?" "I work in the salt mines." This bit of social history could have been very important in this patient's therapy. There he was, working in a salt mine, eating lunch with salt falling all over his food. Perhaps a better initial occupational history would have informed the physician about the contributing factor to the patient's heart failure. According to the professor, stopping work in the salt mines improved his condition.

A senior citizen came under my care for advanced arteriosclerotic heart disease. He had severe angina and took a beta-blocker and nitroglycerin. When I first saw him, he was on the maximum dose of the beta-blocker. His condition resulted in chest pain on walking necessitating a wheel chair. In fact, when I would ask him to get up on the examining table from his chair, he would have to put a nitroglycerin tablet under his tongue to prevent the cardiac pain that would occur just from walking the few feet to the examining table and sitting down. This patient, seen during the early days of cardiac surgery when there were very few medications for this condition, might benefit from the new surgical approach, I thought. I sent him to the local university center. They did a coronary artery angiogram and declared him inoperable. Not dissuaded, I referred him to a cardiac surgery pioneer in another state who happened to be a medical school classmate of mine. He had seven coronary artery bypasses. I saw the patient six weeks later. He said, "Watch me, doc," and took off on a brisk walk up and down my office corridor. This man was a widower, and he surprised me with his next request. "I've got a favor to ask, doc." "What's that?" I asked. "I want you to send me to a urologist," he declared. "Oh, what's wrong?" I asked. "Nothing, I want to get a penile implant." Taken aback, I said, "But, you just had major heart surgery." After amazed contemplation about the miracle wrought by modern medicine, I also said, "Don't tell me you've got a girlfriend already." "No," he said, "but I'm going to get one!"

A sixty-year-old man and his wife went on vacation to the South Pacific islands. They relaxed on the beach, communed with the locals, and enjoyed the exotic foods. When they returned home, diarrhea developed associated with flatulence and cramping abdominal pain. They attributed the symptoms to "changing diets," and decided to wait a while until their "intestinal tract readjusted." However, it did not. When seen in the office, their only physical finding was some upper abdominal tenderness. Stool cultures demonstrated an intestinal protozoa known as Entamoeba histolytica. Proper medication therapy resolved their problem.

Many years ago, a middle-aged woman and her husband were involved in an automobile accident. The woman complained of back pain. X-rays were normal. Sent home, her back pain improved. One week later, she collapsed. The diagnosis—ruptured spleen. She lost considerable blood and had emergency surgery to remove the ruptured spleen. She required several blood transfusions and made an uneventful recovery. Years later, I saw her in my office for the first time. Her current chief complaint was "weakness and loss of appetite." She told me about her accident and the resulting surgery and blood transfusions. This brought to mind the possibility of chronic hepatitis because of the fact that she received the transfusions prior to the time that blood was tested for viruses. The physical examination was unremarkable, but the blood tests showed some abnormal liver enzymes. A hepatitis test proved that she had hepatitis C. On occasion, hepatitis C can resolve, but of all the varieties of hepatitis, hepatitis C has a seventy-five percent rate of chronicity. In some patients, it can lead to liver failure and liver cancer, but that did not happen to this patient.

A middle-aged woman was under my care for vitamin B12 deficiency resulting in a severe anemia. She also had hypothyroidism. She was well controlled. I saw her every six months in follow up. These two problems are autoimmune illnesses, an immune system gone awry attacking parts of the body it suddenly believes are foreign. In the first instance, the body fails to absorb B12, resulting in decreased and abnormal blood production, and in the second instance the thyroid gland fails to make an adequate supply of thyroid hormone. By providing the patient with monthly B12 injections and oral thyroid hormone replacement, the patient is well—not cured—but well. If one has to come down with an autoimmune disease, choose one of these. However, as is often the case, if a patient has one autoimmune disease, they can be prone to getting another. That is why I was very worried when I received a call from her telling me that she had developed shortness of breath, and wanted to see me right away. When she came to the office, her examination was unchanged from previous exams with the exception of perhaps some decreased breath sounds in her lungs. A chest X-ray revealed a condition called pulmonary fibrosis, also known as interstitial lung disease. This is an autoimmune disease where the lung scars over, but it is nowhere near as amenable to therapy as her other two treatable autoimmune illnesses. Cortisone relieved her symptoms, but she experienced a slow and progressive downhill course.

A sixty plus year old physician became short of breath. Examination revealed a loud cardiac murmur. A chest X-ray showed a large tumor in the center of his chest. The tumor put pressure on the heart, caused the murmur and compromised cardiac function. Surgical biopsy proved the tumor to be a very rare and malignant tumor of the thymus gland. The thymus gland is important in immunity, is prominent at birth, and shrinks as one gets older. In the long history of the Mayo Clinic, at that time they had seventeen cases in their registry.

When I was a resident at Cook County Hospital, the evenings I was not on call, I did some moonlighting at a local clinic. The neighborhood I worked in was a less affluent part of the city. On one occasion, an eighteen year old came to the clinic complaining of a "yellowish urethral discharge." Yes, those were his exact words when I elicited his chief complaint. This was enough for me to pay strict attention, because the descriptions I would often get for this particular chief complaint were words not found in Webster's dictionary. Yes, he had made his own diagnosis, describing it as gonorrhea as opposed to the "clap" of his peers. When I lectured him on safe sex, his vocabulary stunned me. For a moment, I thought I was on the Harvard University campus. Penicillin cured him. So I was surprised when he showed up again a month later—yes, you guessed it—with the same diagnosis. This time we extended our conversation, and I suggested to him that he needed to make some better choices. He agreed, admitting that the women whom he was associating were prone to such diagnosis. I also extended the conversation to suggest that he was of an intellectual bent, and seemed to be intelligent enough that when he completed high school, I hoped he would attend college. "You can be sure of that," he said. Now I know you may not believe me when I tell you I saw him once again—yes, you guessed it—with the same diagnosis. We spoke more, by this time adding to the rapport that we had developed. Skip now six years ahead. Into my office strolls this man, well dressed in a suit and silk tie, cashmere overcoat, immaculate, shoes polished like the military. Yes, it was my old friend. "Just thought I'd say hello, doc." We spoke for a while and he took me outside to see his brand new Cadillac parked in the parking lot. "I did what you told me, doc." Smiling, I said, "I'm really glad you came to see me. I'm proud of you. Thanks for coming." He nodded and said, "Uhh—I got a problem, doc." Yes, you guessed it!

A middle-aged healthy man injured his shoulder. He was experiencing considerable pain. His wife had severe rheumatoid arthritis and used a prescribed non-steroidal anti-inflammatory medicine. I forget the exact name of the powerful one she was taking, but the more familiar and milder ones in this family of medications are Motrin or Advil. He came to the hospital emergency room. His chief complaint was weakness, loss of appetite, nausea and vomiting. He felt he was "dehydrated" and it dawned upon him that he had not passed any urine for "a while." When asked if he was on any medicines, he said no, but his wife pointed out that he had taken "one of my rheumatoid arthritis pills for his shoulder." Blood studies revealed evidence of uremia—kidney failure otherwise known as renal failure or renal shutdown. Then the significance of his uremia became evident; he had developed acute renal failure from taking *one* of his wife's pills. What happened to this man was a rare, but known, complication of the non-steroidal class of drugs—kidney shutdown. He had to undergo acute renal dialysis treatments, and made a full recovery.

A twenty some year old Spanish-speaking woman developed severe vaginal bleeding. She spoke very little English, but did manage a chief complaint of "My boy-fren gooz me wid fonnypaper." "What did you say?" a friend of mine, and fellow intern, asked. She repeated her chief complaint. Not understanding what she meant, he placed her on the examining table, examined her and diagnosed the problem. Her chief complaint was accurate. In an attempt to abort his girlfriend's early pregnancy, her boyfriend had rolled up the Chicago Tribune's comic pages into a firm rod and inserted it into her vagina thinking he could end the pregnancy. All he accomplished was a severe vaginal laceration, which my friend sutured. This occurred in the days before Roe V. Wade when potassium permanganate was a favorite method for inducing abortions. This method was by far the most common, and the most dangerous. It was either self-induced or friend assisted. Misusing this toxic chemical is dangerous, as I found out when a patient developed shock. She had placed potassium permanganate directly in her vagina and succeeded in destroying her pelvis including her bladder, and some intra-abdominal intestinal contents. She did not survive emergency surgery.

During my internship at Cook County Hospital, I delivered a twenty-two year old of a healthy seven pound girl—her eleventh child. She informed me that with all her pregnancies and breast feedings she had never had a menstrual period. She did, however, understand the reason why.

A patient asked me if I would see his mother. She was an eighty-six year old resident of a nursing home, and he said he "was watching her deteriorate, and I want to be sure that everything is being done for her." He was willing to bring her to my office in a wheel chair. Her diagnosis was Alzheimer's disease. I told him I would be happy to see her, but I did not want to build up false hopes because there was very little to offer an Alzheimer's patient in those days. She was a tiny woman with thin, sparse white hair and what I am sure would have been beautiful, sparkling blue eyes many years ago. She sat in the wheel chair with head and upper body stooped over. When I said hello to her, she lifted up her head. It was like watching a movie run in slow motion. Her word or words were unintelligible. Her voice was very hoarse and she sounded like a creaking frog. Her skin was dry and flaking, and her reflexes demonstrated a phenomenon known as delayed relaxation phase. When you strike with a reflex hammer—take the biceps reflex for example—the arm should jerk up and down in an equal and rapid manner. In the patient's case, the arm jumped up in a quick, normal fashion, but the down phase was very slow, described as delayed relaxation phase of the deep tendon reflex. All these physical findings were characteristic of an underactive thyroid gland in the extreme, known as myxedema, and unless treated would lead to coma and death. Thyroid replacement therapy—a very tiny dose at first with slight increases every three weeks resulted in improvement over time with increasing strength and mental capability. She lived for four more years and was able to communicate much better with her family.

A thirty-six year old woman developed hypertension in her last month of pregnancy. She delivered a healthy girl, but her high blood pressure did not resolve, so she embarked upon a long quest to get her blood pressure under control. She experienced intermittent success, but more often than not, her blood pressure remained elevated in spite of a wide variety of medications that were tried, and in spite of embarking upon a vigorous exercise program, including many ten and fifteen kilometer races coupled with a thirty seven pound weight loss. The patient also had a serum potassium level lower than normal. The combination of resistant hypertension and low blood potassium should have alerted her doctors to a major problem, but they attributed this combination more to a side effect of the medicines than anything else. The patient did her own Google searches and learned that when a blood pressure is not under control in spite of intensive therapy, it brings to mind several rare illnesses. Life style changes and/or medications taken by a cooperative patient will control at least eighty to ninety percent of high blood pressure. Google went on to tell her that a blood pressure elevation with low potassium demands a careful search for two different types of adrenal gland tumors. She convinced her doctors to order the tests. They did, and unequivocal test results gave the patient no satisfaction because the lab personnel had found an unlabeled twenty-four hour urine sample and "assumed it was hers." Needless to say, this made her angry and over the next year, her physician repeated the tests, but the results were still "not enough for anyone to make a firm diagnosis." She even saw an endocrinologist who told her she did not have an adrenal gland problem. The patient persisted, however, and then, after begging for a referral from her HMO doctor, was sent to a cardiologist who ordered an MRI scan of the adrenal glands, and there they were, not one—but two adrenal tumors (adenomas)! This started her on a search for the appropriate therapy, including seeing a world authority from the University of Oklahoma, and I will not go into the incredible details of all the surgical options open to her, but there was one medical option available. After much soul-searching and personal research, she chose to take a forty-year-old medicine that would block the excess hormone that her adrenal tumors were pouring out and that caused the potassium loss and hypertension. Taking the medication has resulted in a normal blood pressure and serum potassium. This is a perfect example of a patient taking charge of her healthcare! With the healthcare changes to come, much more of such patient take-charge behavior will have to be the norm.

A middle-aged woman came to my office for the first time. She had recently moved to the area where I practiced. Her chief complaint was leukemia. "Who's been taking care of you," I asked. She named doctors at a local university. "Are you on therapy now?" I asked. "No, I'm fine." "Are you in remission?" "If that's what you want to call it, but I've been okay for seven years." I gave her a complete examination and there were no abnormal findings including a palpable spleen (enlarged spleen) that she claimed she "once had." I said, "I would like to get some blood tests and a blood count, and we'll have you sign for us to get a copy of your records." She agreed. The patient's current blood count and all her blood tests were normal. There was no sign of leukemia. The records arrived; yes, they proved leukemia and her physicians at the time treated her. The bone marrow study at the time was confirmatory for the leukemia diagnosis. In fact, she had the type of leukemia that offered a very poor prognosis, but here she was—ten years after diagnosis, and well. How does one explain this?

I saw an elderly woman at Cook County Hospital's hematology clinic. Her chart was on my desk and was at least four inches thick. "Wow," I said, "you sure have a thick chart." She told me that she had been coming to Cook County for twenty years. "What for?" I asked. "I got cancer of the liver." Since it was not likely that anyone with cancer of the liver would live twenty years in those days, or any days for that matter, I was incredulous to say the least, so I opened up her chart from the beginning—and there it was. In fact, there were sketches of her liver based on the physical examination findings. Physicians who had preceded me in the clinic for the last twenty years signed them. Some of these doctors were now my mentors. These drawings showed the edge of a palpable, very large and knobby liver extending far below her rib cage. The liver is, at best, palpable at about the level of the bottom of the rib cage and is very smooth with a defined sharp edge. A liver filled with large nodules is a cancerous liver until proven otherwise. She did not have the benefit of effective chemotherapy in those days. So what do we have? Could this also be another rare case of spontaneous remission of cancer? When I was in medical school, Dr. Warren Cole, professor of surgery, collected 100 case reports of spontaneous remission of cancer. He wrote a book on the subject, hoping to see if there was some common thread to these cases. There was not, so what do we have? Is it divine intervention? Is it a rejuvenated immune system? Is it both? Is it dietary? Is it spiritual? What is the cellular mechanism involved? We are beginning to learn much about these questions.

Rather than give a clinical example here, I will discuss some interesting facts about allergies. They are extremely common. In the United States, fifteen million people suffer from hay fever, ten million have asthma, and even more are allergic to medications, food and insects. Allergies have a hereditary component. An allergy occurs when the immune system overreacts to a usually harmless substance known as an allergen. This allergen enters one's body by a number of routes including the skin, nose, lung and digestive tract. Examples of an allergen are dust, mold, pollen, dander, mites, feathers, foods, drugs and insect stings. This reaction between an allergen and the immune system causes the allergic symptoms. Allergic diseases include asthma, hay fever, hives, skin rashes and insect stings. The symptoms of these illnesses vary from mild to life threatening. Anaphylaxis is the worst allergic manifestation and includes hives, swelling of the throat, breathing difficulty and a sudden drop in blood pressure.

A seventy plus year old man was seen with a chief complaint of urinary difficulty. He did not empty his bladder; he was awakened three or four times per night to urinate and his urinary stream was narrow and slow. As part of his musculoskeletal system review, the patient complained of aching and stiffness of both thighs and hips that was worse in the morning, and improved as the day wore on. He suddenly developed urinary obstruction requiring hospitalization. An urologist performed prostate surgery to relieve the blockage. While in the hospital, a blood count showed slight anemia. This finding, taken together with his morning hip stiffness, raised the possibility of a disorder known as polymyalgia rheumatica. A sedimentation rate 400% higher than normal proved the diagnosis. The cause of the disorder is unknown. It responds to therapy with low dose cortisone. This is another example of a secondary diagnosis resulting from a well-taken system review.

A middle-aged overweight woman complained of severe back pain. It had reached the point where the pain became persistent and varied with position. She could not lie flat or on her back and right side, and was only able to sleep in a reclining position. A complete physical examination was negative except for a retracted area of the skin of the right breast. Obesity prevented adequate palpation of the breast. A mammography proved cancer and a widespread metastasis of the spine was seen on spine X-rays.

I received a phone call from a patient who advised me that paramedics transported his unconscious wife to the hospital. I didn't know his wife, so I was unfamiliar with her medical history. When I saw her, she was immobile, could not move her arms or legs or any other part of her body except her eyes. She had retained cognitive function and responded to questions by blinking her eyes. That was the only part of her face and body that could move. I called a neurologist to see the patient who diagnosed a stroke—located in the pons, an area in the brain stem that relays messages between the cerebral cortex, the cerebellum and the spinal cord. This clinical syndrome, known as the locked-in- syndrome, means the patient, locked in to her own body is immobile except for her eyes. I asked the consulting neurologist, "What's the prognosis?" He answered, "She'll never recover and most patients do not live more than a month." Then he shook his head and said, "If that ever happens to me, be kind and do away with me." The patient remained in the hospital for about two weeks, and then went to a nursing home for further supportive care. Now, as Paul Harvey used to say, comes the rest of the story. This patient made a miraculous recovery to the point of regaining upper body and extremity motion and speech. She progressed to a wheel chair and took her place again on the board of directors of a major Chicago corporation where she had served before her illness. So much for dogmatic medical prognostication.

A middle-aged woman complained of "drooping eyelid and double vision." In addition she noted that after walking, her legs would "get weak, but after I stop and rest they get stronger." These eye and leg symptoms would at times occur together. This is a typical collection of symptoms for a specific neurological illness known as Myasthenia Gravis. It is another in the family of auto-immune illnesses, in this case caused by destruction of chemical receptors on nerve junctions resulting in disruption of nerve impulses. A neurologist confirmed the diagnosis and the patient was started on a drug called pyridostigmine, which again, as in most autoimmune diseases, is not curative, but offers partial to good symptomatic relief.

This report may be familiar to those who read this entire book:

Parents who fled the pogroms in czarist Russian controlled Pale of Settlement, a geographic region where the government required Jews to live, arrived with their four-month-old daughter in the United States on February of 1904. She grew up in the United States, at first living in Rochester, New York and then Chicago, Illinois. She completed two years of High School with very high grades. "You could take two or four years of High School, and I went in the line where my girlfriends were and it turned out to be the two year line." After completing the two years, she went to work as a legal stenographer. She was so good that the lawyers she worked for said that she knew more than they did. In her early twenties, she married a plumber. "I didn't love him, but my father, who knew his father in the old country, liked him and said he was a good man." Family members related that as a young woman, she "saw snakes" and 'acted funny.' She also mentioned that as a young woman, she believes she saw God, a man in a flowing white gown and a long white beard standing at the edge of her bed. She also experienced bouts of depression. She had a son diagnosed as a "blue baby," the name given to congenital cardiac defects for which nothing could be done then. He died in a few days. Her second son was born and thrived. By the time he was a toddler, her mental state deteriorated and required hospitalization for depression. She described this experience as "horrible." "They tied me to the bed. I saw a flame leave my body. It was my soul. I have no soul. How can one live without a soul?

How do you die if you already lost your soul?" I do not believe anyone made a firm diagnosis in those days, and she went home to her toddler son who had forgotten who she was, and a family, including a mother and father, two sisters and a brother, all of whom did not know how to cope. In addition, she now felt in some way contaminated by the experience, and would not touch anybody or anything in the house with bare hands including her own son. All this for fear of bringing upon them the curse that had inflicted her. Her husband could not cope with her illness and left. They were divorced five years later. The relationship with her family deteriorated, the household became dysfunctional and bitter arguments ensued as the family had great difficulty in understanding her bizarre behavior. Her son grew up in this environment, and he too could not understand his mother who refused to ever touch or hug him. If her son tried to hug his mother, she would cry out in anguish and flee. Nevertheless, she was able to go back to work as a legal stenographer, and boarded in her parent's home with her son. She did well at work, was very popular with the attorneys who vied for her services, and who labeled her "the queen of LaSalle Street." At home, however, conditions remained unchanged. She continued to experience intermittent bouts of depression, but never any more hallucinatory symptoms. One bout of depression, later in life, required electroconvulsive shock treatments. Her parents died, her son left home, and she spent her older years living alone in an apartment. She worked until her seventies, all the while her idiosyncracies never changed. She spent the last eight years of her life in a nursing home, visited every week by a daughter-in-law, every other week by her son and at times by her grandchildren and great grandchildren. In her late eighties, she began to develop symptoms of dementia, and as these symptoms progressed, her idiosyncracies regressed, so that by the time she died at age ninety-two she had been able to hold her son's hand and hug him without a single bit of panic or concern.

For many years, I took care of a man and wife. On occasion, they would bring their teen-aged daughter to see me for self-limited minor illnesses such as sore throats or upper respiratory infections. The young woman had no medical problems requiring chronic care. She was tall, attractive, quiet and reserved. When she graduated high school, I was told by her mother that "she's off to college," and at another time, "she's doing well except she's having boy trouble." The last report I received was that she is "living with her boyfriend out of state." Years later, I received a call from her mother asking that I see her daughter, because she had broken up with her boyfriend and arrived home very depressed. When she came to the office with her parents, it was clear that her mother had made the right diagnosis. One could have made that diagnosis from her appearance alone. For want of a better term, she looked miserable. She had a very gloomy affect, a fixed pessimistic, humorless expression, slumped posture, was lethargic and did not make eye contact. She was withdrawn and melancholic. She answered most of my questions by responses such as, "Does it matter?" "Who cares?" "What's the difference?" I completed the interview with a feeling of dread, and I asked her if it would be okay to speak with her parents? "Whatever you want," she responded in a monotone. I brought her parents into another office and told them that I agreed with them that their daughter was very depressed, so much so that I would want her to either be seen by a psychiatrist on an urgent basis, or even better, let me call one of them and make arrangements for her to be hospitalized, because I felt that she was at risk. They informed me that that is what they had wanted for her, but she had refused. She did however agree to see me when her parents offered that option. I told them that I would see what I can do and I went back to speak to the patient. She refused any intervention by a psychiatrist in spite of her not denying that she was depressed. I ended up negotiating back and forth, and the best we could come up with was that I would start her on an antidepressant and the parents, who were both reliable people, would watch her and report her progress or lack of same. I wrote down the name and telephone numbers of two psychiatrists if she changed her mind. One week later, I received a call from the mother. Her daughter had killed herself.That was a shattering experience. Could I have done more? I am haunted to this day.

Although I have given my two examples under the psychiatric history, I must relate one more as an illustration of towering emotional strength that has remained a stirring model for me.

I never saw this elderly woman without a smile on her face. In all the years I took care of her, and in the face of severe symptoms that worsened as she got older, I only received one answer when I asked her how she felt. "Just fine, doctor." Now it was clear that her multiple illnesses made it impossible for her to feel so well, but that is all I ever heard. She would answer yes to specific questioning about pain, weakness, and shortness of breath, but the bottom line to her was that she was "just fine." This never changed throughout the years that I took care of her, even when she progressed into advanced congestive heart failure and developed severe breathing difficulty that resisted all my efforts and the efforts of a prominent consulting cardiologist who hospitalized her for end-stage aggressive treatment. No one was able to understand what kept her going—but I think I knew the answer. In what turned out to be her last hospitalization and while lapsing in and out of coma, she opened her eyes, smiled at me, and moved her hand in a feeble wave. I knew what I would hear when I asked it, but I did anyhow. "How are you?" I said. "Just fine, doctor." she whispered. In addition, in that statement was the secret of her living much longer than anyone would have anticipated. She never perceived herself as sick, or if she did, she never wanted her family to perceive it. She could only think of herself as well, and she did so until the last minute of her life, which gave out at age eighty-four. She was and is a model that I hope I could be able to emulate.

A friend of mine called me on the phone one day when I was making patient rounds in the hospital. He told me about a good friend of his who was ill and getting worse in spite of medical attention. "He's weak and got a fever that won't quit. They told him he has the flu, but I think it's lasting too long." "Yes, I'd be happy to see him," I said, "bring him to the outpatient department." The man was in his fifties, well dressed with suit and tie and a full head of black hair. The patient's vital signs were normal except for a borderline elevated pulse rate of 100 and a temperature of 100.4. Another positive physical finding was an audible cardiac murmur picked up by stethoscope. This was not enough to make a diagnosis, because one could see many patients who happen to have fever from a flu virus and a long-standing murmur that has nothing to do with the flu. However, the decisive factor resided in the patient's fingernails. He had splinter hemorrhages under his nails. These are long thin lines of blood visible on the nail. This unusual finding is diagnostic for subacute bacterial endocarditis, a serious bacterial infection of a heart valve—fatal if left untreated. The combination of the murmur, fever and splinter hemorrhages raised a strong index of suspicion. His blood culture was positive for bacteria, and this was enough to prove the diagnosis. I called a physician that I knew at the hospital the patient lived near and made arrangements to hospitalize him. He responded to massive doses of penicillin for six weeks. When deemed bacteria free, he underwent open-heart valvular surgery and made an uneventful recovery. Though treated with penicillin and blood cultures were free of bacteria, when the surgeons removed his diseased damaged heart valve and replaced it with a new valve, the old valve still grew out some of the organisms. This shows how resistant to medical therapy some of these infections can be. The patient made a full recovery and did well.

A man in his late twenties came to the office with the chief complaint of a "changing mole." The mole was located on the lateral right shoulder area overlying the upper deltoid muscle. It measured one and one half centimeters, was very dark brown with areas of black that he had recently noted. The borders had become irregular and the mole had elevated "higher than it was." He had the mole since he was a teenager, but noticed the change and was aware of the "warning signs." The lesion was consistent with a melanoma, and he went to a surgeon. The surgeon made a wide incision, removed the lesion and confirmed the diagnosis. This young man, the son of a friend, is now middle aged and is well. He gets yearly skin examinations from the surgeon, and avoids the sun or uses sunscreen if he cannot.

I worked at Cook County Hospital as an attending physician on one of the male medicine wards. The responsibility of an attending physician was to see problem patients with the residents and interns and offer advice. I arrived on the floor and went to see a patient who had an enlarged liver and spleen and whose diagnosis was obscure. On the way to see him, we walked by an older man sitting in a wheelchair. The patient had a shaggy white beard and disheveled grey hair—what there was of it. He was wearing a white gown opened in the back and was staring straight ahead with such a doleful expression that I could not help but stop and ask the group about the patient. "Oh, he's just waiting for nursing home placement," said one of the residents. "What's wrong with him?" I asked. "He's senile," one of the interns replied. I asked, "Who saw him first? Did anyone get a history?" "I saw him," said the intern. "No one was with him. The police found him and brought him here. He couldn't answer any questions. He was confused, so we weren't able to get a history. That's all we know." It became apparent to me that the doctors established a diagnosis without the rudiments of a good physical examination for there was a clinical finding that anyone could observe, but had been missed or ignored. I hoped not the latter. This is one of the dangers in a large city hospital that receives patients through the emergency room at a rapid rate and sometimes overwhelms the medical profession by sheer force of numbers. I can remember the times when I was an intern and would admit and work-up a dozen patients a shift. This patient had one pupil much larger than the other. A slight difference in pupil size can be a normal variant—but not this amount of size difference. This finding is an important neurological sign, especially when the enlarged pupil did not react to light by constricting. I asked that they all take a close look. When they did, I also suggested an immediate neurosurgical consultation, because this patient must have sustained a head injury and was suffering from a subdural hematoma, which is an accumulation of blood under the outer lining over the brain known as the dura matter. As the blood continues to leak, the hematoma enlarges, presses on the brain and could cause death if not surgically removed. To make a long story short, they confirmed the diagnosis, performed surgery and the patient improved. The residents and interns learned a lesson. No one will ever be mistake free in this profession. It is reasonable to assume that they will not ignore or fail to evaluate pupil size in a confused man again. In addition, another aspect to that lesson is that doctors are human, and like other humans *can* make a bad judgment—and that is why every patient, if they are able, must be involved in directing their healthcare.

I saw a middle-aged man for the first time when he came to my office for a pre-employment physical examination. He was in excellent health and passed the physical, except for one finding that I could not explain. I held up my ophthalmoscope and said, "Has anyone ever looked into your eyes like I did with this instrument?" He shook his head and said, "I don't remember anyone doing that?" "Is your vision okay?" I asked. "I have no problem," he answered. "Did you ever wear glasses?" I asked. "No, did you see something wrong in there?" "Yes, I did," I told him, "but frankly I don't know what it is I'm looking at. Let me run a quick check of your vision." I took him into another room, and he passed the Snellen chart easily—20/20 in both eyes. "No problem," I said." "Whatever you have there hasn't interfered with your vision and won't interfere with your work, but since I've never seen it before I would like you to see an eye doctor, just to be sure it's nothing significant." He agreed. What I saw was two irregular rounded, small, pure white spots lying on the peripheral retina. The patient did visit an ophthalmologist, and was diagnosed histoplasmosis of the eye, or "histo spots." Histoplasmosis is a fungus, known as histoplasma capsulatum, found in the dust and soil, mostly around the Mississippi and Ohio rivers. Studies have shown that the majority of adults living in the area are carriers. They have inhaled the spores dropped on the dirt by birds and bats. After a person inhales the spores, they can end up anywhere in the body, but the body's immune system prevents this. However, the spore does have a tendency to find the eye where, out of the soil and in an adequate environment, it activates and causes disease. If the patient is unlucky, the spore will end up in the central retina where it could cause a blind spot. On inhalation of the spores, some do get a mild flu like illness that is transient and passed off as "a virus." Those with a compromised immune system could get a full-blown systemic case involving multiple organs. I saw a few more histo spots during the rest of my career, but on those occasions, I could make my own diagnosis. And that is why there is nothing like time, careful examinations and experience to enhance one's skills.

A middle-aged man came to my office with the chief complaint of "I can feel a little lump in my ear. When I put my little finger in my ear to scratch it, I can feel the lump." I confirmed his finding. He had a typically appearing basal cell carcinoma in the ear canal, a rounded lesion with heaped up edges and a central depression. This is a very slow growing malignancy that can be destructive at the site, but metastases are rare. He underwent Mohs microscopic controlled surgery. The surgeon incises tissue borders until the specimens removed are determined to be tumor free by a pathologist who evaluates the specimens with a high-powered microscope. The patient is many years past the procedure and has no recurrence in the ear, although follow up examinations have revealed other sites where basal cell carcinomas have formed.

Sometimes patients can take charge of their health to such an extent that they do not need physicians anymore—at least in the early stages of their medical interaction. A young woman patient called me for referral to an ear doctor. As an HMO member, she required a referral from her primary care doctor. She said that she was losing her hearing and she was sure she was getting otosclerosis. Otosclerosis is a degeneration of the bones in the middle ear to the extent that the bones become spongy resulting in fixation of one of the three tiny bones in the middle ear, the stapes. This, in turn, prevents the bone from vibrating, and therefore the sound does not transmit to the brain. Why do you think you've got otosclerosis?" I asked. "My mother has it," she said, "and the same thing is happening to me that happened to her. She had to have surgery." Now that is a precise and to the point medical history and she received the ear specialist referral via this phone message. The patient called the office of the ear specialist and spoke to his nurse, inquiring as to the physician's experience in performing stapedectomy—a surgical procedure where an artificial prosthesis replaces the non-vibrating stapes bone. She learned that the physician did not perform stapedectomy, but his nurse gave her the name of a doctor who does. At this point, she was getting frustrated with the system, so she talked to the HMO medical director, explaining to him that she was certain of her diagnosis, she had already saved them money by not going to the ear doctor's office. So, why not just let her go to the office of the doctor who performs stapedectomy, since he had the most experience in performing the tests to determine what option was best for the patient: stapedectomy or medical therapy using fluoride and a hearing aid. By this time she knew all there was to know about the disease. For sure, she knew more than I did. The medical director agreed, and she saw the specialist who did perform a stapedectomy. She is in the running for the take-charge patient of the year award.

A man in his mid-thirties came to see me for an upper respiratory infection. On examination, I discovered a large round defect in his nasal septum. It was, I would estimate, about a centimeter in diameter. In zeroing in on this part of his medical history, I asked him if he had had nasal surgery. The answer was no. Likewise was the response to questions about trauma, chronic nose picking, cortisone nasal spray use, exposure to toxins, nose ring and a list of rare problems that might cause a nasal septal defect. This left cocaine use as the remaining etiology that I could think of—to which he confessed.

My wife and I received an invitation to dinner at our neighbor's house. There we met a man and wife, friends of our neighbor. When the man found out I was a physician, the conversation turned to the state of his medical health—as it so often does. For a year, he had experienced nasal symptoms including bloody and purulent nasal discharge. He saw his physician on many occasions and, as he stated, his doctor found that his sinuses were tender and there were "sores" in his nose. Therapy would result in improvement, but the symptoms would recur. On another occasion, his physician treated him for an ear infection and pneumonia. To make a long story short, nothing that the doctor could do would result in a permanent cure. His nasal symptoms worsened. This failure to improve prompted a visit to see an ear nose and throat physician whose nurse took the history. "Do you see many patients like me?" my new friend asked the nurse. "No, not many, but enough so that I'm quite sure I know what's wrong." The patient's eyes lit up. "What is it?" he asked. "I'll let the doctor see you," she answered. "He should be here in just a few minutes." The patient had developed an unusual condition known as Wegener's granulomatosis. This is an autoimmune disease that causes inflammation of the upper, and sometimes lower respiratory tract. It is an inflammation of blood vessels, which starts in the nasal area and may spread to the lungs and kidneys. The prognosis for this disease has improved with the use of immunosuppressive agents and cortisone. We saw this man again five years later at the fiftieth wedding anniversary party of our neighbors who had moved out of state. He was free of disease and feeling well.

A middle-aged woman complained of a "lump" in front of her right ear. She had at first "felt something the size of a pea," but noted that it was increasing in size. When I saw her, she had a firm, non-tender, movable lump. There were no other abnormal findings. A plastic surgeon removed a benign parotid gland tumor known as a mixed tumor.

An elderly male smoker complained of "white spots in my mouth that I can't scrape away." Examination revealed small, white deposits (leukoplakia) resulting from chronic irritation of the mouth due to smoking. He was a smoker for fifty-five years, and had never before been able to stop, so I urged him again to stop smoking, and sent him to an oral surgeon for reinforcement—if nothing else. The condition may turn cancerous if the patient keeps smoking, but it can resolve if the patient stops smoking.

A senior citizen presented with a small plum sized mass above the clavicle on the right side. The initial impression was that this mass was an enlarged lymph node. It was non-tender, firm and fixed in location. The patient underwent a complete physical examination, and there were two smaller lumps adjacent to the larger one. There were also enlarged lymph nodes in the chest as shown by CT scan. Surgery demonstrated that the plum sized mass was a Non-Hodgkin's lymphoma of a particularly aggressive variety. The patient underwent surgery, radiation and chemotherapy. He has remained free of disease.

A teenaged boy developed an enlarged lymph node on the right side of his neck. Examination revealed it to be firm, non-tender, movable, and two and a half by one and a half centimeters. He told me that it had been there about two weeks. There were no other lymph glands palpable, and scalp, ear, nose, throat and mouth examination were normal. I recommended removal if it did not show decrease in size in the next two weeks. His sister, a nurse, did not want to wait another week or two and took him to see a surgeon who excised the node. There was no malignancy. The pathologist felt that it was a "reactive benign node" perhaps from some recent local infection.

A middle-aged woman had a chief complaint of shortness of breath, especially with exertion. She also complained of awakening from sleep very short of breath. This is due to left-sided heart failure (failure of the left ventricle). Examination of her heart revealed a soft blowing systolic murmur, and what I interpreted as a gallop rhythm (instead of a lub dub there is a lubdub-dup). The murmur was maximal in intensity near the apex, or bottom of the heart and suggested the diagnosis of mitral insufficiency. In other words, the mitral valve did not close well when her left ventricle beat; therefore some of the blood ejected from the left ventricle, instead of going to the aorta through the aortic valve, leaked back through the damaged mitral valve into the left atrium. There are a number of causes for this incomplete closure of the valve, and they are an enlarged left ventricle, which stretches the valve, and rheumatic fever that can damage the valve. However, I didn't expect to find what the echocardiogram identified—a left atrial myxoma, a benign and rare cardiac tumor. Surgery was curative.

As an intern, I admitted a patient to the hospital for fever, weight loss, night sweats and a chronic productive cough. Our initial presumptive diagnosis was tuberculosis. On the day of admission, a much older attending physician came to Cook County to make rounds with us. This physician had an excellent reputation as an outstanding diagnostician. We looked forward to his visits. It seemed to us that there was nothing that this man did

not know. He was a superb teacher. He had been practicing almost fifty years, and trained in the early twenti-
eth century including a few years in Vienna—if memory
serves me—at the Allgemiene Krankenhaus. Rumor had
it he would wake up every morning at five o'clock to
study the latest medical literature. It was the custom to
present each case by giving the full medical history,
which we provided to this esteemed physician. He asked
the patient to sit up in bed with legs over the side. The
physician then took up a position facing the patient's
back and proceeded to percuss his lung fields. This
seemed to take an unusual amount of time, and when he
finished, he said to us, "Come closer and bring a pen."
We did. "Watch and listen," he said, and he percussed
the patient's posterior chest and every few seconds he
would stop and make a mark on the patient's skin. We
listened and watched as he percussed from right to left
and left to right, from up to down and down to up. When
he finished he had a well-defined ten by twelve centimeter oval marked out on the patient's posterior, upper
chest. He said, "I agree with your diagnosis of tuberculosis, but I think you'll also find that this patient has a
tubercular lung abscess located here." We all looked at
each other in amazement, for this was a remarkable
achievement. No one else in that room—or any room for
that matter could equal it. An X-ray of the chest confirmed the abscess just at the precise location where the
physician had percussed it out on the patient's chest.
This physician received his medical education when
William Konrad Roentgen discovered X-rays. Physicians trained in that era had nothing to go on except their
own senses, so they developed them to a physical diagnostic capability we will never equal in the modern
high-tech physician.

A young man came to Cook County Hospital complaining of shortness of breath. Examination of the lungs

demonstrated the following on the right side: observation—no unusual findings; palpation—no findings; percussion—loud, hollow sound (from escaped air in chest cage); tactile fremitus (a feeling of vibration) absent (from collapsed lung no longer adjacent to chest wall); auscultation—no breath sounds due to lung collapse. This man had the classical findings of a pneumothorax—air escaping from the lung into the chest cavity. The air pressure in the chest cavity results in a lung collapse—either partial or complete. Pneumothorax can result from trauma, but there was no history of it in this case. He had a spontaneous pneumothorax, caused by a ruptured air cyst on the lung. This is one of the easier diagnoses to make based on physical examination findings if the doctor takes the time to do it carefully. An X-ray confirmed the diagnosis, and told us the extent of the pneumothorax.

A middle-aged man developed sudden onset of severe abdominal pain. In order to walk he had to stoop forward and clutch his abdomen. He had never experienced such intense pain before. His physical examination demonstrated marked left lower quadrant tenderness, including rebound tenderness (pain after sudden release of the examiners hand after pressing down on the abdomen). When he lay on his back he kept his knees up, which helped relieve some of the discomfort he was experiencing. There was distention of his abdomen and diminished bowel sounds. A rectal examination was uncomfortable for the patient, but there was no blood or any masses palpable. He had a low-grade fever and an elevated white blood cell count. An X-ray of the abdomen showed air under the diaphragm. This meant that the patient experienced a gastrointestinal tract perforation with the escape of air from his intestine into the abdominal cavity. The location of the positive abdominal tenderness suggested the possibility of a perforation of a colon diverticulum, or a perforated malignancy. Surgery revealed a perforated diverticulum. The surgeon resected (removed) a short segment of the colon and sewed the ends together. The patient did well.

A diabetic patient was under good control taking oral diabetic medication. He watched his diet, lost twenty pounds and was doing well. I saw him every three months on follow up visits. On one occasion, he came to the office at his wife's insistence, because she thought the whites of his eyes had turned yellow. She was correct. His skin was also becoming yellow. A urinalysis demonstrated dark urine and a rectal examination showed light colored stool on the examining finger. The patient developed obstructive jaundice. Something was blocking the entry of bile into the intestines. He had no pain whatsoever, a silent jaundice, and one of the main causes is cancer of the pancreas, which this patient did indeed have. It was inoperable. He knew what lie in store for him, and he chose to put all his affairs in order. To do this gave him great comfort in what was to be his remaining few weeks.

A patient of mine brought her husband to see me. He was complaining of severe back pain due to recently diagnosed Paget's disease. This is a disorder of bone where the normal turnover of old bone cells being replaced by new is accelerated in certain localized areas. Softened and enlarged bone replaces the normal bone matrix. The X-ray picture shows increased bone whiteness, coarseness and thickening. In spite of symptomatic attempts at pain relief, his pain worsened. I examined the patient, and the main physical finding was on his rectal examination. His prostate gland was enlarged, irregular and hard. It had several easily palpable, rock hard, one to two centimeter nodules. This was diagnostic for prostate cancer and a prostate specific antigen test of over two thousand was confirmatory. The normal prostate specific antigen test is under four, although one could have cancer even with a normal PSA. This patient had advanced prostate cancer with metastasis to the bone. Paget's disease can mimic this X-ray picture. He underwent orchiectomy, a surgical removal of the testicles, and sees an oncologist for chemotherapy. He had instant relief lasting for two years until the disease reasserted itself and spread to his liver.

A middle-aged woman had hypertension. As part of the physical examination, I thought I could palpate a mass in the patient's right upper abdominal quadrant under the liver. "Yes, I sometimes have some discomfort there," she said. I ordered a scan of the abdomen and it showed a very large kidney cyst. Since she had few and mild symptoms, and the cyst did not demonstrate any findings suggesting malignancy, a urologist is following it by physical exams and ultrasound to determine if there are any changes suggesting a trend toward malignant degeneration, a rare, but possible result.

When I completed my internship at Cook County Hospital there was no chance to start a residency, because there was a doctor draft in place and we were all committed to spend two years in the military. This was a known and expected interlude to what already was a long educational experience. We spent six weeks training at Fort Sam Houston, Texas, and then received our duty assignment. Mine was the 101st airborne division at Fort Campbell, Kentucky. During our orientation, the chief of service, an obstetrician, asked his new medical recruits, "Who among you have delivered babies?" Four of us raised our hands. "How many?" he asked. Since my volume was close to two hundred deliveries more than my closest competitor, the chief, a lieutenant colonel, said, "Okay Captain Cohen, you're on OB call.

You'll work with me today and start call tomorrow." Like any good soldier, all I could say was "Yes sir." In the time spent at Fort Campbell, I added a considerable number of deliveries to my total, and learned an important lesson that I have never forgotten. I saw a young woman in the gynecology clinic who complained of pelvic pain. The pain was sudden in onset and accompanied by some vaginal spotting. Her vital signs were unremarkable. I performed a pelvic examination and found her to have tenderness and pain on cervix movement. My initial impression was pelvic inflammatory disease (PID), a diagnosis made many times at Cook County Hospital. I told the commander about the case and my diagnosis. He said, "Did she miss any periods?" "Uh-h—I forgot to ask," I answered. He asked the patient, and she had. He examined her, turned to me, and said, "This lady has an ectopic pregnancy." She went promptly to surgery for her fallopian tube pregnancy. Yes, my chief was right. This was a humbling and important lesson for me. Never forget to take an adequate history.

A classmate of mine saw a patient in his office. Her chief complaint was a vaginal discharge. My friend, a family practitioner who was brand new in practice, examined the patient and confirmed the presence of a purulent (pus) vaginal discharge. On speculum examination, he discovered the cause—a foreign body was present, and this set up the infection. The foreign body turned out to be a condom. Now the rest of this story should have never happened, but it did, and no doubt speaks to inexperience. My friend reassured the patient's husband that his wife had developed an infection because of a condom left in her vagina, and that they both needed to be more careful and make sure that they do not forget the condom in the heat of passion. The husband's response—"Doctor, I don't use condoms."

On a routine follow-up examination of a female diabetic patient, she told me that she was experiencing dull and aching pain in her right shoulder. She also said that the movement of her shoulder was becoming more difficult as time went on. She had some localized tenderness along the upper shoulder and upper arm. Her range of motion was limited. She could not remember any recent trauma to her shoulder. I was not sure why she was having this difficulty, but I recommended she see an orthopedic surgeon. The orthopedist made a diagnosis of "frozen shoulder." Why it happens, no one is sure, but it does occur more frequently in diabetics. The capsule of the shoulder gets inflamed and thickened and freezes up. He prescribed anti-inflammatory medications, heat and physical therapy including stretching and range of motion exercises. He reserved the use of cortisone injections if this initial therapy was not enough. The illness does get better in time.

As an intern at Cook County Hospital, I saw a young man in the orthopedic clinic who had injured his right arm. Physical examination revealed a deformity of his right upper arm. It was severely swollen, black, blue, and very tender. The deformity was located about six inches from the top of his shoulder. An X-ray revealed a complete break of the humerus with the bone separated and angled at the fracture line. The orthopedist told me to put on a hanging arm cast with a sling. This is a cast from the shoulder to the wrist with the elbow bent at a right angle. The theory is that the heavy cast pulls the bone into place and it will heal in about six weeks. The patient received post-cast instructions and I told him to return to the clinic in three weeks. When I saw him three weeks later he seemed fine except for one thing—he wasn't wearing a cast! "What happened to the cast?" I asked. "When I left here last time I had to play a basketball game, so I cut off the cast," he answered. Amazed, I asked, "Did you put it back on?" "No," he smiled. I shook my head in disbelief. An X-ray showed perfect healing with a straight humerus and solid new bone formation. Mother Nature is still the best healer!

During my intern days at Cook County Hospital, I spent a month on the neurology service. There were a number of patients who lived on the ward. They had unusual neurological symptoms and physical findings, and they were teaching examples for medical students, interns, and residents. One cooperative patient had a classical syndrome. His neurological examination revealed findings localized to the lower extremities. His lower legs were weak. Patellar and Achilles tendon reflexes were absent. He could not feel a vibrating tuning fork touching his shins. When you moved his toes up or down with his eyes closed, he did not know in which direction you moved them. He failed the knee to heel test, his heel falling off his lower leg when trying to slowly move his foot from the knee to the ankle. He did not feel pinpricks on his legs and his Romberg sign was positive...that is when he stood upright with his eyes open, he had no trouble standing, but when he closed his eyes, he would lose his balance. Patients can stand with eyes closed and not lose balance, because they can feel sensations from the bottom of their feet and know where they are. They also know where they are because of vision. In the case of this patient, he lost the ability to know where he was because of the pathology of his legs and feet, but he could keep his balance if his eyes were open. When he closed his eyes, however, he lost both the eye and foot neurological sensory mechanisms, and since he had nothing to tell him where he was, he would lose his balance. With all these abnormal neurological findings, it was clear that this patient lost the use of the posterior columns in his spinal cord. And he lost them because of destruction by syphilis—a condition known as tabes dorsalis—which manifests itself about twenty to thirty years after the initial infection.

A "droopy eyelid" was the chief complaint of a middle-aged man who came to my office. A droopy eyelid is termed ptosis. On examination, his right eyelid almost completely obscured his vision on the right and he could not raise the eyelid by willing himself to do so (ptosis). I examined him and found that the pupil on the right side was much smaller than the left (miosis). Clinically, it was clear that the patient had ptosis and miosis involving the right eye. This is two thirds of a triad of symptoms, the third one being anhidrosis, an absence of sweating of the face on the same side. I asked him if he noticed this symptom, but he was not sure. I had seen him during the winter months. The neurological findings of ptosis, miosis and anhidrosis are a characteristic triad known as Horner's syndrome, caused by an interruption of the autonomic sympathetic nerve supply to the eye. This interruption can result from a stroke, or by a malignant tumor on the very top of the lung known as a pancoast tumor. Because the patient had been a smoker for many years, this was my first thought. A chest X-ray confirmed this impression.

I am reminded of a patient who was about to undergo elective surgery. This woman had a list of questions for her anesthesiologist. I know her well, and she is the type of person who receives comfort based upon full disclosure and knowledge of what she is about to face, good or bad. She and Google are on intimate terms. She met her anesthesiologist for the first time the morning of surgery. He introduced himself, took a brief history, listened to her heart and lungs and reviewed her chart. When he completed this quick introduction, the patient told him that she had a list of questions for him. "How many?" he said. The patient held up a sheet of paper with about ten written questions. "About ten," was the reply. "I'll answer three," he said with an impatient look on his face. The shattered patient got her three questions answered, but then went into surgery depressed and scared. Such pre-operative preparation is not conducive to good outcomes. This is a proven fact, and sure enough, this patient had a stormy postoperative course. Later she confided in me and told me the whole story. "It made me angry at the whole medical profession," she said. I suggested to her that at that time she should have taken charge of her health. She should have told the anesthesiologist to take the few minutes necessary to answer the questions that were important to her. If he still refused, then she should have told the anesthesiologist that he needed to get in touch with her surgeon, because unless she had the questions answered, she was prepared to refuse to have the surgery performed at this time and in this place, and she would tell the surgeon the reason for her decision and request another anesthesiologist. As you can imagine, most patients are too meek to assert themselves in this manner, but who has more right.

One more example to illustrate a point: I took my competitive swimmer, eleven-year-old grandson, Ethan, to a sports medicine doctor for a painful elbow. The doctor did a very careful exam and diagnosed an injury to the biceps tendon where it inserts on the elbow bone. As part of the exam, he checked the area with a tuning fork. This was something I had never seen before and I asked what he was doing. He told me that if there were a stress fracture, the placing of the tuning fork would cause the patient to not only feel the vibration, but also some pain. Now, I have been a doctor for a long time and I never knew that. I tell this story to illustrate that physicians never stop learning and we discover new things every day.

This completes about all I can remember about my patient care experiences, as you can see, a constant source of education for physicians. This takes us to the next chapter, a painful, but necessary bit of information in relation to the life of a physician—malpractice.

CHAPTER 14
MALPRACTICE

It didn't take long for me to experience this morass and bane of the medical profession. I had just started practice, was still working in an inner city clinic when a process server gave me my gift—a malpractice case against me for the care of an infant patient given penicillin who subsequently had a seizure blamed on the penicillin and required hospitalization. Interesting—internists don't see infants. Someone sued me for another doctor's patient. As it turned out, the final diagnosis was viral encephalitis, but that would hardly negate the lawsuit in this medico-legal environment. The Chicago Cook County attorneys couldn't care less who saw the patient, they routinely sued all the doctors whose name was on the door under the legal theory, "We don't know the relationships of all the doctors in the clinic, so we sue 'em all and sort it out later." Can you imagine the expense? All the doctors received their gift including the psychiatrist, and I personally was present when the process server handed the subpoena to the two dentists who rented space. I still remember the expression on their faces as they stood there, subpoena in hand and mouths agape. I quickly learned that the lawyers sued about 1000 healthcare providers per month in Cook County; an attorney's delight, a physician's nightmare. At least my defense attorney assigned to defend me by my malpractice carrier was a fine man from a prestigious downtown Chicago firm. We would become good friends over the years; he becoming my patient. His son was an orthopedic surgeon friend of mine. This case lasted five years. It took almost that long for all the machinations to occur before the attorneys dropped the physicians from the case. The only ones not dropped were the actual attending doctor and me. Apparently, the plaintiff's attorneys tried to make the case that I, as the first and busiest doctor in the clinic was the, "Boss of the clinic." That was news to me and I emphatically disagreed, but that delayed things for many years as the morass and all the legal mumbo-jumbo continued beyond my ability to comprehend. "Just let me handle it." advised my attorney friend. "You just go on practicing medicine." Much later into the process, I received a call from my attorney who announced that, "We decided that rather than go on with this nonsense and continued expense, we'd make them go away with a small settlement."

That was my quick introduction to the world of malpractice. A case on my record, settled without my knowledge so it could "go away," and nothing I could do about it. Welcome to the world of malpractice, Sheldon.

Years later, I learned of another lawsuit against me for a patient I never saw. I found out that this patient came to the emergency room apparently for a non-serious medical problem, was treated and released and received my name in follow up because the patient did not have a personal physician and I happened to be the doctor on call in the emergency department for internal medicine that day, a rotating requirement of all doctors on the staff. The patient left the ED, walked to his car and slipped on the ice breaking his shoulder. Brought back in to the ED, they admitted him under the care of an orthopedist. I knew nothing of this interaction until I learned much later that they sued the hospital and me because my name was on the ED record as the "doctor on call." Eventually they dropped me from the suit.

I saw a patient in my office that moved out of Chicago to Elk Grove Village. Her chief complaint was incision pain. Her medical history revealed breast surgery for a very early cancer, and since the surgery, she was experiencing pain. As it turned out, I knew the surgeon from Cook County Hospital, an academically brilliant and technically superb surgeon with an excellent reputation. She currently was not on any further therapy, but the pain was worsening. Since she did not want to go back to Chicago to see her surgeon—she hoped I could "fix it here," I sent her to a local surgeon who did indeed give her relief via a nerve block. She was very satisfied. The malpractice suit followed, involving her original surgeon, me, and the surgeon who gave her relief. She had no knowledge of what her attorney had done and when she found out, she appealed to her attorney to drop me and the surgeon who relieved her pain from the suit. I never heard anything more about it.

I saw a new patient in my office, her chief complaint being fatigue and a rash. A complete physical examination revealed a rash, suspicious in my mind for vasculitis (inflamed blood vessel), an unusual and potentially serious condition. This coupled with an enlarged spleen (a very unusual physical examination finding) raised the suspicion of a serious blood disorder. Initial blood studies were not remarkable except for some abnormal liver function studies that complicated the issue and increased the urgency. My recommendation was to see a hematologist and I sent her to the chief of hematology at a local university who discovered that she had cryoglobulinemia, an abnormal protein, which may or may not be associated with disease including a malignancy, which the hematologist found. The patient died.

It did not take long for her son to hire an attorney who promptly sued the consulting hematologist and the referring physician...me. As it turned out, her son was also a patient of mine, and when I saw him in the office, I asked him if he really meant to sue me? He manifested a shocked impression, said the suit was for the hematologist and apologized, saying that he would, "Tell the lawyer to get me off the suit." It took a year. A sad follow up to this case occurred about two years later when the son came to my office with a rash—vasculitis! Just like his mother! He also had a painful hip and upper leg. Studies revealed the same cryoglobulinemia as his mother had, and X-rays revealed a bone malignancy from which he did not survive.

The last and final case took fifteen-years, and was extremely depressing because it occurred to a very good forty-four-year-old friend of mine who was an employed physician of the hospital. Shortly after I moved in to my hospital medical director office in 1973, he walked in and asked if he could see me on a medical issue. "Of course," I answered. "Let's go to the outpatient department."

He related that last evening he experienced a bout of chest discomfort for the first time. There were no other symptoms and it lasted only a few minutes. He promised his wife he would see me in the morning. I took a history, did a complete medical examination, and an electrocardiogram, all of which were normal. I documented all this on a sheet of typing paper in my medical director's office and placed it in a desk drawer. This would prove to be a critical issue in the future. I ordered a blood profile including cardiac risk factors and ordered an exercise stress test. The blood tests were fine, but no stress test results were forthcoming. "I've got your blood test results, but where's the stress test?" I asked. "Oh, I'm feeling great, so I decided not to do it." I could not talk him out of that stance and advised that the best way to rule out heart disease would be the exercise test, and its absence made the diagnosis now impossible to evaluate. He assured me he was fine. We saw each other almost on a daily basis at the hospital. He never complained of any more symptoms to me. Six weeks after I saw him at the initial examination, his wife called me at 3:00 am and advised that her husband collapsed and was on his way to the hospital via ambulance. He was there when I arrived and I declared him dead. I attended his funeral. The hospital pathologists preferred not to do the autopsy, since the deceased was also their good friend. A neighboring hospital pathologist performed the autopsy. He died of a heart attack, but surprisingly, the pathologist did not find any coronary artery blockage, or so their report stated.

Two years later, process servers did their thing presenting me with a suit on behalf my friend's wife. They also served papers on the hospital and even sued the other hospital where they performed the autopsy. Crushed, I went to get his medical record, but I could not find it! This would come back to haunt me. I was very foolish for not bringing the patient record from the hospital to my private practice office when I initially saw the patient.

The sum demanded in my case—eleven million dollars. I had one million in malpractice coverage supplied by an insurance company that with others would eventually flee the state because of excessive losses. The Illinois State Medical Society filled in the gap and provided insurance rather than have all physicians go bare. It would be a long ten years before the malpractice case came to court. My expert witnesses were two university chiefs of cardiology who testified that I met the standard of care. The plaintiff's expert, a very young new general practitioner, said I should have hospitalized him. After 6 weeks of trial, the jury came in with a ten to two verdict in my favor—a hung jury. Five more years passed and the lawyers argued procedural issues, some of which had to do with my lost record. These issues, in preparation for another trial, apparently prevented my expert witnesses from testifying to certain matters, complicating my case even further—all beyond my comprehension. I had the scary feeling that the plaintiff's attorneys were outsmarting mine.

To make a long story short, I faced, much more than before. At the advice of my attorney, who left the decision to me, I settled for less than my malpractice limits rather than face the risk, no matter how small, of bankruptcy. At least the widow would benefit. As if that wasn't enough, the settlement took place on a date one day after the government ordered mandatory recording of all malpractice settlements in a National Practitioner Data Bank. I must have been one of the first so recorded—for a fifteen-year-old case.

I believe you would agree that these experiences give me some justification for commenting on the malpractice crisis in the United States, The costs are enormous and physicians all practice defensive medicine as a result, further raising costs. The current Affordable Health Care Act (Obama) is silent on the issue of malpractice reform...not a word. I liken it to a lottery with multimillion-dollar awards. I doubt this system will change requiring physicians to continue to practice defensively, keeping costs up. To understand this, let us say that a patient presents with unusual symptoms, and the possible diagnoses include one that has a one in 1000 possibility. The test to make this diagnosis, which has its own risk to perform and costs 4,000 dollars, is the only way to find out. The physician will order it, ignoring the rare possibility, as a protection against a future lawsuit. For in a court of law, the laws of probability will have little relevance to the average jury; the doctor missed the diagnosis by not ordering the test, therefore he or she is liable.

Another reason for the incredible number of medical malpractice cases is the contingency fee system, which allows the filing of any suit; no up-front costs to the plaintiff rewarded when the suit ends with victory—if it does, or in defeat—still no cost to the plaintiff.

In a philosophical bent, let me offer the proposition that the Affordable Care Act is merely a first step of an evolution to a completely socialized medical system to come, patterned after most of the rest of the world where socialized medical systems reign and the great majority of physicians are salaried.

With all the aforementioned in mind, let's discuss the malpractice system in Germany, socialized since the late 1800's. Anyone who feels he or she is a victim of malpractice can approach the doctor or hospital's liability insurer. More often than not, they will reach satisfaction and settle, caring for the injured patient's needs as long as necessary. If the patients do not receive satisfaction at this level, they may approach a medication board free of charge and hope for resolution. Failing this approach in the patients mind, the patient has the option of utilizing the court system if they are willing to risk paying the costs including court costs, the costs of the opponent (hospital or doctor or both), and the winning party's costs. The German government does not allow the contingency system.

Think about this approach. It will be a major topic of discussion the next ten years as our healthcare system transitions.

CHAPTER 15
RETIREMENT

When I was appointed medical director the second time, I left my medical practice association, moved to a solo office for private practice and took on my role as medical director again, only this time under peaceful conditions; the new hospital-physician collaborative model of medical care accepted, not only at Alexian Brothers, but also around the country. At this point, I hoped I could devote a good five years to this task and then retire. My children were married and gainfully employed; my wife, who acquired her nursing master's degree with honors, became Director of Nursing Education at a Chicago hospital. I assumed my new duties, worked an intensive five years and then retired after selling my medical practice in 1994, my wife having retired after about fifteen years on her job. We would spend a few years traveling, something we always dreamed of doing, but before I get into more retirement activities, let me tell of an interlude involving a personal health matter.

When I was about fifty years of age, I vowed to return to physical activity from the couch-potato existence I had been accustomed to living with. With this in mind, I started a jogging routine and worked my way up to 5, 10, and 12K races. As I improved, on one occasion while running indoors on an oval track, I started a sprint. When I ran around the curve rapidly, I felt a pain and "tear" under my left armpit. The next day, I could not use my left hand. I discovered this when my hand did not have the strength to turn a door knob, making me realize how weak it was. This lasted a few days and the strength returned. Obviously, I injured (tore) the nerves going from my spine to my left arm. Since I recovered full use in two days I forgot about it, except for the fact that over the next years, I would get a rare recurrence of the left arm pain—flare up of the old arm injury, I thought. As it turned, this would be a classic case of denial, because one day, when I was 66 years of age, close to two years after I retired, the left arm pain returned, persisted and worsened. No more flare-up theories—this is probably cardiac, I thought, even though I never experienced chest pain. I saw Dr. James Mason, cardiologist at the hospital, now named the Alexian Brother's Medical Center, and he confirmed my suspicions. My coronary angiography demonstrated one coronary artery with a major block and three other minor blocks, all bypassed by Dr. Sullivan a Loyola trained cardiovascular surgeon. I may well owe my life to Dr. Mason who diagnosed my case and Dr, Sullivan who performed the surgery. My postoperative course was uneventful and the doctor discharged me in four days. I would be one of the about twenty percent of patients who go on to develop a post cardiotomy syndrome, or Dressler's syndrome, named after Dr. Dressler who described it years ago in patients following a heart attack that involves the pericardium. Since heart surgery also involves cutting the pericardium (outer heart lining), Dressler's syndrome can also occur after heart surgery. It is an autoimmune pericardial process characterized by typical pericardial pain. I had 7 progressively diminishing attacks over four years, as best as I can tell, a record period of time. It was more of a nuisance than painful. Here I am sixteen years later without a symptom and with normal cardiovascular risk factors. I owe much to my two superb physicians.

So what did I do in retirement. First, I joined the complete physical examination program offered at the hospital. Two mornings per week, I saw two patients each time who wanted to avail themselves of a complete examination. I emphasize the word complete, because the exam took at least an hour including a full history and a complete head to toe physical examination. Putting the results together with basic laboratory studies, we would dictate a comprehensive report of our diagnostic impressions and recommendations for further evaluation if necessary. The patient received the report to take to his or her personal physician.

Second, because of my administrative ten-year experience as medical director of the hospital, plus serving as the initial medical director helping to start two HMOs in the Chicago area, Cigna and Humana, the Joint Commission on Accreditation of Healthcare Organizations offered me a position as a quality consultant. I took this part-time position and very much enjoyed working for two of their divisions, Joint Commission Resources and Joint Commission International. In this capacity, my responsibilities were to assess quality in hospitals throughout the United States and the world. I travelled to Rio De Janeiro, Brazil, Copenhagen, Denmark, and Kiev, Ukraine where besides the hospitals I evaluated in all three locations, I served as a consultant to the Ministry of Health in Ukraine to help them develop standards for a hospital accrediting organization.

After up to six years in these activities, I devoted full attention to my remaining interest in post private practice retirement—writing books. I had an idea for a book, *Brainstorm,* but no time to do any writing while in practice. Now that I had free time, I said to myself, "Start now or forever hold your peace." It was like the blind (me) leading the blind (me), for I did not seek assistance in any manner, and for a guy who hated English courses in school it was more than laughable. It took me four years to come up with a final version. I did give the first draft to a professional for some comment after about a year of writing. She asked, "Is this supposed to be a novel?" "Yes," I replied. She countered, "It's a fine medical report, but it's no novel." She proceeded to write me several pages of advice.

Back to the drawing board, I went. After four more drafts, I was ready to take the literary world by storm. I found a literary agent who accepted my work. I didn't realize, at the time, that she was brand new to the agency business and had very few clients. Soon she announced that she had acquired a publisher for the book, but I would have to pay to get the book published. What did I know? In my anxiety, I agreed. The small publishing house in California in business for thirty-five years and not a self-publishing operation, which meant they did not charge fees, (that should have been a wake-up call for me, but I was too naïve) took on my project, managed to print about two-hundred of my books and promptly declared bankruptcy. The only good news is that Amazon still lists the book. I did get the few books the publisher printed and stored them away as a reminder of my folly. Where Amazon would get any to sell, I have no idea. Welcome to the publishing business, Sheldon. I recently published a new electronic version of *Brainstorm.*

I did continue to self-publish the rest of the books I wrote and electronically published more. It remains a wonderful hobby and I credit writing, healthy eating, and walking a dog a mile or two a day with keeping this elderly brain and body intact.

CHAPTER 16
MEDICINE 1951-2012

Consider this chapter a medical educational experience. It is 61 years since I started on a medical career, and the practice of medicine today bears no resemblance to what it was when I entered medical school. In contemplating the state of medicine in 1951, the advances are breathtaking, not to mention what is on the drawing board for the future. With this in mind, I would like to put on paper my perceptions of the state of the art in 1951, and its evolution by 2012. Being an internist, I will zero in on internal medical issues.

The most fascinating educational experiences for me as a student, intern, and resident were the clinical pathological conferences already mentioned in a prior chapter of this book. A physician received the medical records of an undiagnosed patient who died and had an autopsy performed. The records did not include the autopsy report with its final diagnosis, and the presenting physician would present the case discussing the history, physical exam, laboratory and X-ray studies, and give a diagnostic impression to an eager audience in a large auditorium trying to do the same from their progressively rising semicircular rows of seats surrounding the lecturer. The majority of the time, lecturers would hit the nail on the head, but when they missed, livelier discussions ensued. Many of these cases had to do with diseases of unknown etiology at the time, mostly autoimmune diseases, and this brings me to my first topic: the immune system and autoimmune diseases taken from my book The Slim Book of Health Pearls: MAN THE BARRICADES: THE STORY OF THE IMMUNE SYSTEM.

THE IMMUNE SYSTEM AND AUTOIMMUNE DISEASE

The immune system is a fascinating story about the body's defenses against attack by enemies constantly trying to harm us. The principal actors are organs, cells, and complicated collections of proteins, tuned by billions of years of evolution to work in a harmonious manner for the good of the whole. These principle actors keep us alive in a world where, on a daily basis, invisible or visible predators want to usurp our bodies. These predators are bacteria, fungi, pollen, viruses, parasites, and cancer cells. In the face of this onslaught, we owe a state of good health to our immune system: the collaborative mechanism that protects us from disease by utilizing a sophisticated team of specialized organs and cells that differentiate self from non-self. This ability stems from the fact that every body cell carries distinctive molecules (epitopes) on their surfaces that identify it as self. Immune cells, recognizing this self-marker, coexist peacefully in a state known as self-tolerance. On the other hand, altered or foreign cells or organisms that do not carry this self-marker will find themselves subjected to a vigorous assault by the immune system.

It's a battle to the death. The rules of war are—take no prisoners; kill or be killed. That is how the immune system functions in defense of life; how human beings stay alive. The cells and structures of the immune system are the body's razor-edge trained military. They have taken an oath to protect the body that gave them life, and they carry out that oath pre-programmed with a single-minded purpose: kill the invader. When they function as programmed, human beings stay safe. When they weaken, humans may die.

The principle cells of the immune system that kill invaders are lymphocytes, a type of white blood cell that circulates in the blood stream. Different lymphocytes have different appearances under the microscope, and in 1951 when I asked my professor why there were different types of lymphocytes, his answer was, "I have no idea." Such was the state of knowledge of the intricate cellular working of the immune system in 1951. Now, in 2012, we know exactly what each lymphocyte does.

Before staring on the topic of autoimmune diseases, an historical perspective is important. A medical student sixty years ago learned about a multitude of diseases. With great assurance, professors would lecture about the symptom complexes making up a specific disease, the patients history of the onset of the disease, the manifestations of a full blown case, the physical findings related to the disease, the laboratory findings indicating the presence of the disease, the expected clinical course of the disease, the pathologic findings, the therapy, if any, and the autopsy findings. Once medical students digested these hundreds of different diseases, hopefully they took their place in a long line of diagnosticians and healers. I use the word healers with tongue in cheek for there was not much healing going on; symptomatic relief, yes, rarely full healing.

The answer to the question, "What causes it" was "We don't know." Or if the professor had a humorous bent the answer would be that the disease is a member of the family of GOK'S disease."

"And what is that?"

"God only knows."

We now know that most of those diseases fall into the category of "autoimmune disease," defined as a disorder in which the body's immune system mistakenly identifies normal cells as abnormal, attacking them and causing injury. Although there are no outright cures for most autoimmune diseases there are therapeutic interventions that make it possible for many people to live symptom reduced normal lives if they stay under frequent medical surveillance.

Millions of people are affected by autoimmune diseases; women more than men. They are affected during their working and childbearing years. For some unknown reason minority groups are involved to a greater degree. For example, Lupus Erythematosis is more common in African-American and Spanish women.

Autoimmune diseases are diagnosed with difficulty and often late because the symptoms, the physical findings and the laboratory results may tell little in the early course of the disease. So it becomes important to follow and monitor the patient. Even this may not lead to a diagnosis as the patient's symptoms may resolve or wax and wane. Physicians may not be able to foresee, based upon the initial symptoms, what the course of the disease will be. Sometimes an incredible amount of patience is required of the physician and the patient before making a definite diagnosis.

Researchers have identified seven different mechanisms causing autoimmune illnesses. They all have to do with conditions in the body that arise at the cellular level causing the lymphocytes to think the cell they are surveying does not belong to "self." Here is a list of 1951 GOK diseases (2012 autoimmune diseases).

AUTOIMMUNE DISEASES BY SYSTEM

Endocrine glands:
Diabetes Mellitus
Hashimoto's Thyroiditis
Grave's disease
Autoimmune oophoritis and orchitis
Addison's disease

Nervous system
Myasthenia Gravis
Multiple Sclerosis
Guillain Barre

Gastrointestinal system
Crohn's disease
Ulcerative colitis
Chronic active hepatitis
Primary biliary cirrhosis

Musculoskeletal system
Rheumatoid Arthritis
Polymyositis

Skin
Psoriasis
Scleroderma
Dermatitis herpetiformis
Pemphigus vulgaris
Vitiligo
Lupus erythematosis

Blood vessels and Heart
Wegener's granulomatosis
Dressler's syndrome

Blood
Hemolytic anemia
Pernicious Anemia
Thrombocytopenia

Urogenital
Glomerulonephritis

Eyes
Sympathetic ophthalmia
Sjogren's syndrome

The attempt to classify many of these probable auto-immune diseases by organ system is an oversimplification, because many of these illnesses involve multiple organs.

In treating autoimmune diseases, the first principle to understand is that they are chronic illnesses requiring a lifetime of monitoring and care. Many of these illnesses are controllable and people can live normal lives. Physicians can cure a few autoimmune diseases even though there is no resolution of the underlying cause. For instance, pernicious anemia was a serious illness that led to death before scientists discovered the cause— B12 deficiency. Using as little as a monthly injection of B12 cures the patient. Physicians have done nothing to the underlying disease process. They have given the victim of the autoimmunity the substance that the autoimmune process has prevented the body from utilizing.

Stress is the next topic I would like to discuss (Taken from my book, The Slim Book of Health Pearls: HORMONES NERVES AND STRESS).

STRESS

Never taught as a separate course in medical school, stress was only mentioned on occasion. In the 1950's, physicians were researching its ramifications and slowly coming to conclusions concerning its importance. Hans Selye, the stress pioneer, a Czechoslovakian physician working in Canada during the 1930's, accidently discovered it as a potent force in physiology and medicine. Slowly and surely, Selye and others worked out the physiological prime movers in the stress reaction: the endocrine system and the autonomic nervous system, that branch of the nervous system that functions beyond conscious control.

In 1951, physicians had incomplete understanding of the endocrine system.

Endocrine glands produce and secrete hormones into the blood stream to reach their target site of action. Early 1900 physicians and scientists believed that the endocrine glands worked autonomously; each doing its own thing independent of the other, but by the 1950's, they learned that they worked together producing hormones, chemical substances that act on the body to:

1. Direct the body's metabolism (all the body's physical and chemical processes)

2. Regulate body growth, sexual development and functioning

3. Assist in the coordination of the functions of different parts of the body

The known glands, their hormones, and their "autonomous" function at that time were as follows:

- Thyroid gland: secretes hormones that regulate body metabolism

- Parathyroid gland: four embedded in the thyroid gland regulate calcium levels in the blood and bone

- Reproductive glands (ovaries and testes) responsible for the sex hormones that produce male characteristics and sperm production, and female characteristics, egg production, menstruation, and pregnancy

And with the most relevance to our study of stress the

- <u>Adrenal glands</u> These glands (two…each one perched on top of the kidneys) are triangular shaped glands composed of two parts:

  1. The outer part known as the adrenal cortex produces hormones called glucocorticoids (cortisol), which regulates the body's metabolism, salt and water metabolism, the immune system (not well understood in the 1950's and also plays a part in sexual function…and

  2. The inner part known as the adrenal medulla produces epinephrine (adrenalin), which helps the body confront physical and emotional stress by increasing blood pressure and heart rate and force.

The adrenal glands play the major role in the stress reaction.

Also, by the 1950's, physicians understood that the pituitary gland was the master gland, the conductor of the endocrine symphony orchestra whose hormones controlled all the other endocrine glands, telling them when to carry out their physiological effects. Since the pituitary, a pea-sized structure encased in a protective bony cocoon known as the sella turcica, hangs from a portion of the brain known as the hypothalamus at the base of the brain...what is its connection to the brain? Since we are but a brain and the rest of our body's purpose is to keep our brain (us) alive...there must be a connection, and since that part of the brain that the pituitary hangs from is the hypothalamus, does the hypothalamus exert some control of the pituitary? Does it elaborate some hormones that could control the pituitary just as the pituitary controls the other endocrine glands? If so, how do these hormones selectively get from the hypothalamus to the pituitary to exert their effect?

Hormones from the endocrine glands travel through the blood stream to reach their end-target and exert their effect. Is this how the hypothalamus works as well? The mystery was about to be unraveled, and the unravelers were Roger Guilleman and Andrew V. Schally.

Guillemin was born in Dijon, France and graduated as a physician in 1949. In the 1950's he went to the University of Montreal, studied with Hans Selye and received a Ph.D. in physiology in 1953. Following this, he joined the Baylor University College of Medicine where he worked until 1970.

Schally, born in Wilno, Poland, now Vilnius, Lithuania, received a Ph.D. in biochemistry from McGill University and then joined the Baylor University faculty where he worked in conjunction with Guilleman until they separated and moved to other universities. They did, however, continue their collaboration trying to unravel the mystery of the hypothalamus.

Their intense efforts succeeded and they shared the 1977 Nobel Prize in Physiology or Medicine for "for their discovery concerning the peptide hormone production of the brain." The pieces had all fallen into place. How does this work? The hypothalamic hormones travel the very short distance down nerves and capillaries to the pituitary. What are these hypothalamic hormones and what are their effects?

- Thyrotropin-releasing hormone (TRH)

  Causes the pituitary gland to release thyroid stimulating hormone that will stimulate the thyroid to release its hormones to affect metabolic activity.

- Prolactin-releasing hormone (PRH) and Prolactin release-inhibiting hormone (PIH)

  These two hormones stimulates the pituitary to release prolactin which causes lactation

- Gonadotrophin-releasing hormone (GnRH)

  Stimulates the pituitary to release follicle stimulating hormone that stimulates the testes to produce testosterone and the ovaries to produce estrogen

- Growth hormone-releasing hormone (GHRH) and Somastatin (SS)

  These two hormones affect the release of growth hormone by the pituitary

- Corticotrophin-releasing hormone (CRH)

  Stimulates the pituitary to release adrenocorticotrophic hormone, which will cause the adrenal glands to liberate cortisol and epinephrine

The latter (CRH) has the most relevance to the stress response.

HYPOTHALAMIC>PITUITARY>ADRENAL AXIS is the vital endocrine part involved in the stress response.

Now that we've brought the hypothalamus into the picture, let's get into its function in a little more detail.

The hypothalamus is that portion of the brain responsible for homeostasis, from the Greek homeo meaning the same, and stasis meaning stable. Recently, scientists have replaced the word homeostasis with allostasis from the Greek word allo meaning "variable," suggesting that there is some variability in baseline stability, thus "remaining stable by being variable." Allostatic regulation brings cephalic (brain) regulation into the mix to accept the variability of baseline stability. In keeping with this current concept, the author will switch to the word allostasis.

The body strives to maintain stability. It does this by adjusting to changing conditions in order to keep a uniform internal state of balance. The hypothalamus of the brain is responsible for maintaining allostasis. Think of it as a thermostat, which allows control of home temperatures. The difference is that a home thermostat controls only temperature while the hypothalamus controls numerous physiological processes to keep the body in a constant state of equilibrium. It does this by reading changes in a variable that should be held at as constant a level as possible and making adjustments if necessary.

For instance, to assist in the regulation of blood pressure, stretch-sensitive cells in the neck arteries carrying blood from the heart to the brain are stimulated if the blood pressure elevates. This stimulation sends a message to the hypothalamus, which then stimulates the vagus nerve causing the heart to beat more slowly decreasing blood pressure.

A decrease in blood volume due to reduction in blood plasma, the liquid portion of the blood, occurs from dehydration and brain sensors detect this and stimulate secretion of substances that causes contraction of tiny blood vessels (arterioles) leading to the blood capillaries. This arteriolar contraction reduces the flow of blood into the capillaries thus reducing pressure making it possible for fluid in the intracellular spaces to migrate back into the capillaries restoring blood volume. In a similar manner, cell sensors within the hypothalamus read body temperature. If too high, the hypothalamus initiates heat loss through sweating and opening up skin blood vessels to bring increased blood flow to the skin for heat evaporation.

The hypothalamus, links the nervous system to the endocrine system (neuroendocrine function) via the pituitary gland allowing control of internal body organs to maintain a state of allostasis that functions automatically beyond conscious control.

This completes the discussion of number one, the endocrine system, so now we will discuss number two, the nervous system and its collaborative role with the endocrine system in the stress response. The nervous system is composed of three parts:

1. Central nervous system includes the spinal cord and the brain.

2. The peripheral nervous system includes twelve pairs of cranial nerves that originate in the brain. They direct muscular movements of the head and neck and receive sensations from the head and neck. It also includes thirty-one spinal nerves that control body and extremity muscular movement, and receive sensations from the periphery that travels through the spinal cord to the brain.

3. Autonomic nervous system is beyond our conscious control: heartbeat, blood flow, breathing, digestion.

The brain's outer layer is the cerebral cortex. The cortex is composed of two halves: right and left—known as the right cerebral hemisphere, and the left cerebral hemisphere. The cerebral cortex is the sight of intellect. It is responsible for insight, thought, memory and reasoning. Both cerebral hemispheres have four lobes, each responsible for specific functions. These are:

1. Frontal lobe (front portion)—personality, intellect and emotions.

2. Parietal lobe (rear-top portion)—sensation.

3. Occipital lobe (rear-lower portion)—sight.

4. Temporal lobe (side portions)—hearing and speech.

The cerebellum is another part of the brain, separate and below the cerebral cortex. It is responsible for coordinating complex muscular movements such as running, walking, swimming, and playing a musical instrument. The cerebellum operates with no conscious control.

The basal ganglia are nerve bands buried deep within both cerebral hemispheres. They control automatic associated body movements.

The thalamus acts as a relay station between the spine and the cerebral cortex where the nerve cells, known as neurons, meet. This meeting site is known as a synapse, and it acts as a relay station that delivers impulses to the periphery from the brain and to the brain from the periphery.

The brain stem is a connecting nerve link from the spinal cord to the brain. It is composed of three parts where nerve tracts ascend and descend. It is also responsible for automatic control of respiration, heart and gastrointestinal function.

The spinal cord occupies the upper seventy percent of the bony vertebral canal. It consists of long nerve tracts that start in the periphery from the skin, muscles, tendons, and internal organs, enter the spinal cord, and reach their final destination in the brain. These nerve tracts, known as sensory pathways, deliver sensations of hot and cold, touch, pain, pressure and vibration. In addition, they also act as motor pathways delivering messages from the brain to the periphery that control purposeful movements.

This completes a broad overview of the nervous system.

Following is a discussion of the autonomic nervous system that together with the endocrine system constitutes the two major mechanisms controlling the stress response. The autonomic nervous system's main function, through its innervation of all body organs autonomously and continuously without conscious input, controls all the neurological and endocrine (neuroendocrine) functions of the body for the purpose of maintaining allostasis.

The best way to understand this is by example, but before giving an example, it would be important to know that there are two parts of the autonomic nervous system: the sympathetic and the parasympathetic branches.

The sympathetic nervous system prepares the body for intense emotion and extreme exercise (fight or flight).

The parasympathetic nervous system conserves energy and brings the body back to a restful state.

In general, the autonomic nervous system consists of nerves that run between the central nervous system (hypothalamus) and various internal organs...those beyond our conscious control. These internal organs and their response to autonomic control are:

	SYMPATHETIC	PARASYMPATHETIC
• Pupils of the eyes	Constricts	Dilates
• Salivary glands	Stimulates flow	Inhibits flow
• Gastrointestinal tract	Stimulates peristalsis and secretion	Inhibits peristalsis and secretion
• Heart	Slows heartbeat	Accelerates
• Blood pressure	Decreases	Increases
• Lungs	Constricts bronchi	Dilates bronchi
• Liver	Releases bile	Converts glycogen to glucose
• Urinary bladder	Controls	Involuntary void
• Reproductive glands	Functioning	Shut down
• Growth	Functioning	Shut down
• Immune System	Back to baseline	Increase

With the above endocrine and neurological background in mind, let us experience a stress reaction.

Please pretend you are an antelope strolling in the African grasslands. The grass is tall, juicy and delicious after a recent rain. You stroll along enjoying the meal, thankful for the peace and quiet, the excellent weather and the opportunity to eat your full, satisfying your appetite and using energy for present use and storing energy for the future. Life is good.

Then out of the corner of your eye, you see a crouching lioness in the distant grass, her eyes directly on you! Your head pops up, your body stiffens. What is that lion's intention!? When you suddenly see her leaping forward and running right for you in a full gallop, you understand. Within two seconds, you activate your sympathetic nervous system and deactivate your parasymapathetic nervous system; you stimulate the hypothalamic, pituitary, adrenal axis to liberate cortisol and epinephrine. You are in full fight or flight mode. What happens in the next minute or so will determine whether you live or die. You flee for your life. This double rapid activation of the neuroendocrine system is your only chance.

Let's break it down into different actions although they all happen simultaneously within seconds:

1. The light bouncing off the lion's body enters your eyes aided by the rapid pupil dilation allowing you more direct sight and travels through the optic nerve to the occipital cortex where it is turned into the lion's image allowing you to "see".

2. Your entire brain, activated, recognizes that you are no physical match for the hungry, rampaging lion, so you choose the flight part of the fight or flight response, and activate the hypothalamus turning on the sympathetic nervous system and the pituitary and the adrenal glands to elaborate cortisol and epinephrine so as to enhance the physiology giving you your only chance of escape. Your neuroendocrine system has heard the bugle call and acted immediately.

3. Your pupils dilate in response to the sympathetic nervous system's order. After all, fleeing for your life demands sharp, distinct, broadened vision to help you run while keeping your eye on the fast running lion and evaluating the best route of escape.

4. Before you saw that lion, your digestive tract was in full operating mode to take care of all that delicious grass for current and future energy needs. The instant you saw her, you sent a sympathetic nervous system directive to desist immediately. This turns off saliva (have you ever had a sudden dry mouth at the onset of sudden stress?), and slows down stomach and intestinal tract peristalsis and digestive enzyme secretion. After all, there is something more important going on now and you need all your energy to promote the necessary physiological actions that

may save your life. Assuming you survive, you'll activate your parasympathetic later and restart your digestive processes.

5. Since you are going to be running for your life, your thigh muscles are going to need all the blood they can get. The muscles will be more active than they have ever been, so the demand for blood with its life saving glucose and oxygen is critical. Therefore, your heart is called upon to furnish more blood to these active muscles, and through your neuroendo-crine system (sympathetic nerves, and epinephrine elaborated by the adrenal cortex), the heart speeds up and the blood pressure rises; all this in an effort to fulfill the need for an enhanced blood supply to your running muscles to try to keep you from being the lioness' next meal.

6. While you were grazing on the delicious grass, and in the recent past, you had plenty to eat. In fact, you took in enough carbohydrate to allow you to meet the current need for energy plus allow you to store the excess in the liver as a substance called glyco-gen. Since you need all the energy you can get in this life and death emergency, your neuroendocrine system will pull out glycogen and turn it back to glucose for instant energy use.

7. In this critical time, you have no need for functions such as growth and reproduction. Shut those down. You'll turn them on later—assuming there is a later.

8. Platelets circulate in the blood. They are cellular-like structures that function to assist blood clotting. While you are in this fight or flight mode, you could suffer serious bloody injuries. You need all the means available to stem bleeding. Make as many platelets as you can.

9. Fleeing for your life, as well as the chance that you can lose some blood, may dehydrate you. Calling on the pituitary to release anti-diuretic hormone will prevent the kidneys from allowing plasma water excretion in the urine. This will conserve fluids and keep the blood fluid volume up.

10. Since you are in this fight or flight mode, there is a possibility that you will receive a lacerating, contaminated injury with invasion by bacteria and foreign bodies, so you need to enhance your immune system to be better able to confront these invaders.

This completes the "fight or flight" response. In this case, stress is good; it is the only chance to save your life.

The lion caused the antelope extreme stress. Hopefully, you have a better understanding of the physiologic mechanisms called into play; the autonomic nervous system and cortisol and epinephrine.

If the antelope escaped and the lion walked away, the antelope will relax, its parasympathetic will reactivate, reestablishing allostasis.

As best as we can understand, animal's stress is isolated to these life-threatening events. Unlike humans, they do not have financial troubles, junior is not into drugs, they don't have a mortgage to pay, they don't get fired or laid off from jobs, they don't worry about a place to stay. Life is simpler. Whether they will be a meal for some predator seems to be their principle concern and as long as that doesn't happen, and their food is plentiful, what else is there that could be stressful for them? Granted, this may be our thinking based upon incomplete knowledge of what goes on in an animal's brain, but what we do know for certain is that human beings have a multitude of thoughts, problems, situations and pressures on an ongoing basis, any one of which could elicit the stress response.

Human beings then can find themselves spurting cortisol and epinephrine in their blood streams on a frequent intermittent basis. Needless to say, this life saving response may be beneficial, but it won't be if it does not get turned off, restoring allostasis. Chronic stress is harmful if repetitive over time, as the examples below illustrate.

Physical stress (exercise) is excellent for a healthy heart, but dangerous for a diseased heart. The decision to embark on an exercise program should only be made after consultation with a physician, because a person who has coronary artery disease with blocked arteries may not be able to meet demands on the cardiac muscle induced by exercise; the heart becomes ischemic (starved of oxygen) resulting in angina (cardiac muscle pain) or a heart attack (death of heart muscle).

Emotional stress is another story. What effect on the heart results from repeated emotional stress, the kind of stress that liberates cortisol and epinephrine and prepares the body for fight or flight? This is a difficult problem to generalize. Stress means different things to different people. What is stress for one may not be stress for the other. How one responds to stress may have more relevance than the stress itself, but enough evidence has surfaced that demonstrates some kinds of emotional stress in some people under certain circumstances may contribute to heart and blood vessel disease and exacerbates already existing disease.

In the modern era, when human beings are under emotional stress, the surge of cortisol and epinephrine results not in fight or flight, but rather in a suppressed, perhaps very relaxed reaction all presented to the outside world through clenched teeth, drawn, suppressed fists and a polite smile.

There is no doubt that internalizing a fight or flight response may be harmful to the heart and vascular system, especially in those who cannot suppress their anger.

What kind of emotional stress in what type of person is bad? It turns out that people who have little control of their lives or work are affected the most by emotional stress, whereas bosses, those who are at the top level of organizations or companies fare much better than their employees. It appears that the sense of control is the key.

This is true for the most part, but the equalizer for every person is the sudden very severe emotional shock that suddenly impacts one; death of a child or spouse, divorce, business failure, outside near death experiences etc. These could impact all alike regardless of social order. Also, the impatient, always on edge, everything is urgent, competitive, angry type of person fares badly to stress as regards coronary artery disease.

The cardiovascular system is the organ system that stress damages more than any other part of the body. By turning on the sympathetic nervous system and turning off the parasympathetic nervous system, by secreting cortisol and epinephrine, the heart rate and blood pressure rises. With chronic stress, that blood pressure progressively increases. As the blood circulates through the blood vessels with more force, the muscle layer in the blood vessel wall enlarges just as any muscle undergoing physical stress. This increases the rigidity of the blood vessels and it therefore takes more and more forceful cardiac pumping to propel the blood. In time, the heart will begin to suffer; it enlarges and weakens.

As the blood vessel musculature enlarges as the blood pressure elevates, the blood vessel gets thicker and more rigid. In response to the increased force and turbulence within the blood vessels, the interior walls may get little tears causing inflammation. This sets the stage for plaque formation, a combination of arterial wall deposits of cholesterol, calcium, inflammatory cells, glucose, and fat. Known as atherosclerosis (hardening of the arteries), this slow, progressively increasing blockage of the blood vessels may result in a heart attack or stroke.

Stress plays a major role in cardiovascular disease, and its role in other areas includes:

- Repeated stress accelerates the aging process
- Repeated stress impacts the immune system and can result in autoimmune disease
- Stress may cause impotence
- Stress is known to cause abortions and makes in vitro fertilization less likely to work
- Chronic severe stress in children may stunt growth
- Chronic stress can cause psychological gastrointestinal disorders
- Stress may cause and can exacerbate depression

On to the next topic:

HYPERTENSION

In 1951, I can recall hearing that treating an elevated blood pressure carried risks because lowering blood pressure could impair blood perfusion of the heart and kidneys, resulting in potential failure of these organs. A second approach disagreed with this concept and attempted to treat elevated blood pressure. There were no anti-hypertensive medications to speak of, although I can remember my grandmother receiving a prescription for phenobarbital (a sedative) because of an elevated blood pressure "over 200," as I recall her saying. I was in medical school at that time and when she arrived home from the doctor with that news, I took her blood pressure and my reading was 110 over 70. She concluded, "You don't know how to take it yet." She was probably a "white coat hypertensive," but I do not believe that was a recognized concept at that time. It may be, however that I inherited that tendency, because while my BP is normal at home, it usually is not at a doctor's office. Regardless, there were those who believed an elevated blood pressure required therapy and championed one of two approaches: The first was the so-called rice diet, a diet consisting principally of fruit and rice (low salt, calories, fat and protein). This caused weight loss and did improve blood pressure in some, but many in the medical community failed to embrace this approach. The second approach, a surgical one, included cutting the sympathetic ganglia in the lower thoracic and upper lumbar area. This approach lower some blood pressures also, but did have a side effect—postural hypertension (fainting when suddenly standing up). At the same time, two medications tried included reserpine and veratrum alkaloids both of which could reduce blood pressure but had significant side effects that caused physicians to abandon their use in some patients. However, by 1952, there were those who championed the idea that any hypertensive patient with good kidney function is a candidate for medical therapy. Thinking turned seriously to medication use for hypertension

By the late 1950's, the thiazide diuretic group of medications demonstrated excellent blood pressure control and represented a true break-through in anti-hypertensive therapy . This opened the door and in the years since the late fifties, four other groups of drugs including beta-blockers, angiotensin-converting-enzyme (ACE) inhibitors, calcium channel blockers, and angiotensin-receptor blockers (ARBs) benefit the great majority of patients with hypertension. Either one drug, or their use in combinations can effectively treat blood pressure for the great majority.

Regardless of these statistics, however, problems remain because many people with hypertension are unaware they have it, and of those who know and are on therapy, many are not well controlled. This represents a failure in the system as a whole and cries out for correction. Normal blood systolic pressure in 1951 was considered to be 100 plus your age. Normal blood pressure in 2012 is 120 to 130 over 80 or less.

This bring us to our next topic

MYOCARDIAL INFARCTION (HEART ATTACK)

The James B. Herrick cardiology award honors a physician who made a significant advance in clinical cardiology practice. James B. Herrick was that physician, the first to diagnose a heart attack on a living patient in 1912. The fifty-five-year-old patient lived fifty-two hours. An autopsy confirmed Herrick's clinical impression that an obstructed coronary artery led to the patient's demise. Physicians, loathe to accept his interpretation, caused Dr. Herrick to comment that his case report, "Fell like a dud." Never the less, slow acceptance finally did elevate Dr. Herrick to a secure place in cardiology history.

Even though this new diagnosis came upon the medical scene, physicians had no therapy to offer. The patient, put to bed, underwent monitoring and lived or died while physicians pontificated. As late as 1958, when I started my internal medicine residency in a geriatric center, one of the attending doctors suffered a heart attack, and I made rounds with the physician assigned to care for him. I stood there and listened as he said, "You've got to be at complete bed rest, and I mean if your nose itches, don't raise your arm to scratch it."

Prolonged bed rest, sedation and oxygen were the main stays of myocardial infarction care. Many were cared for at home. Some physicians advised that recovering patients rest for up to six months. Such was the state of medical care knowledge for heart attacks in 1958 and into the 1960's.

In 2012, heart attack therapy begins even before diagnosis. Today, all physicians, and hopefully most patients are aware of warning signs. Anyone exhibiting these signs and symptoms should seek medical care immediately. Timely diagnosis and treatment with "clot busters," medications such as aspirin, heparin, other antiplatelet drugs or combinations, whose purpose is to break up the artery-blocking clot and minimize heart muscle damage is crucial. At the same time, the use of medications to dilate blood vessels, control pain and guard against the possibility of life-threatening cardiac rhythm disturbances will be part of an initial cardiac regimen.

Since the days of bed rest, cardiac care has become aggressive. Cardiac catheterization laboratories allow the investigation of the coronary arteries before or immediately after symptoms, and if cardiologists find a significant arterial block, they have the options of angioplasty or stents to open up the artery, or coronary artery bypass surgery to restore blood supply to the injured heart—all a far cry from, "You've got to be at complete bed rest, and I mean if your nose itches, don't raise your arm to scratch it."

EPILOGUE

This ends my story and a brief review of a few changes in the practice of medicine from 1951 when my colleagues and I started medical school and today, 2012. The rapidity of the changes makes me feel as if I became a physician in the stone age of medical practice. Staying abreast of these changes is a difficult task for physicians in their own specialty, not to mention the impossible task of staying abreast of all medical specialties. For anyone contemplating a career in medicine, know that you must never let the bad aspects of medical practice interfere with the good you can accomplish while dealing one-on-one with patients in a compassionate and caring manner. There is nothing like it and your reward will be a happy and fulfilling life.

If this book has convinced one reader to pursue a medical career, it will be well worth the time and effort I put into writing it.

Sincerely,

Sheldon Cohen M.D. FACP

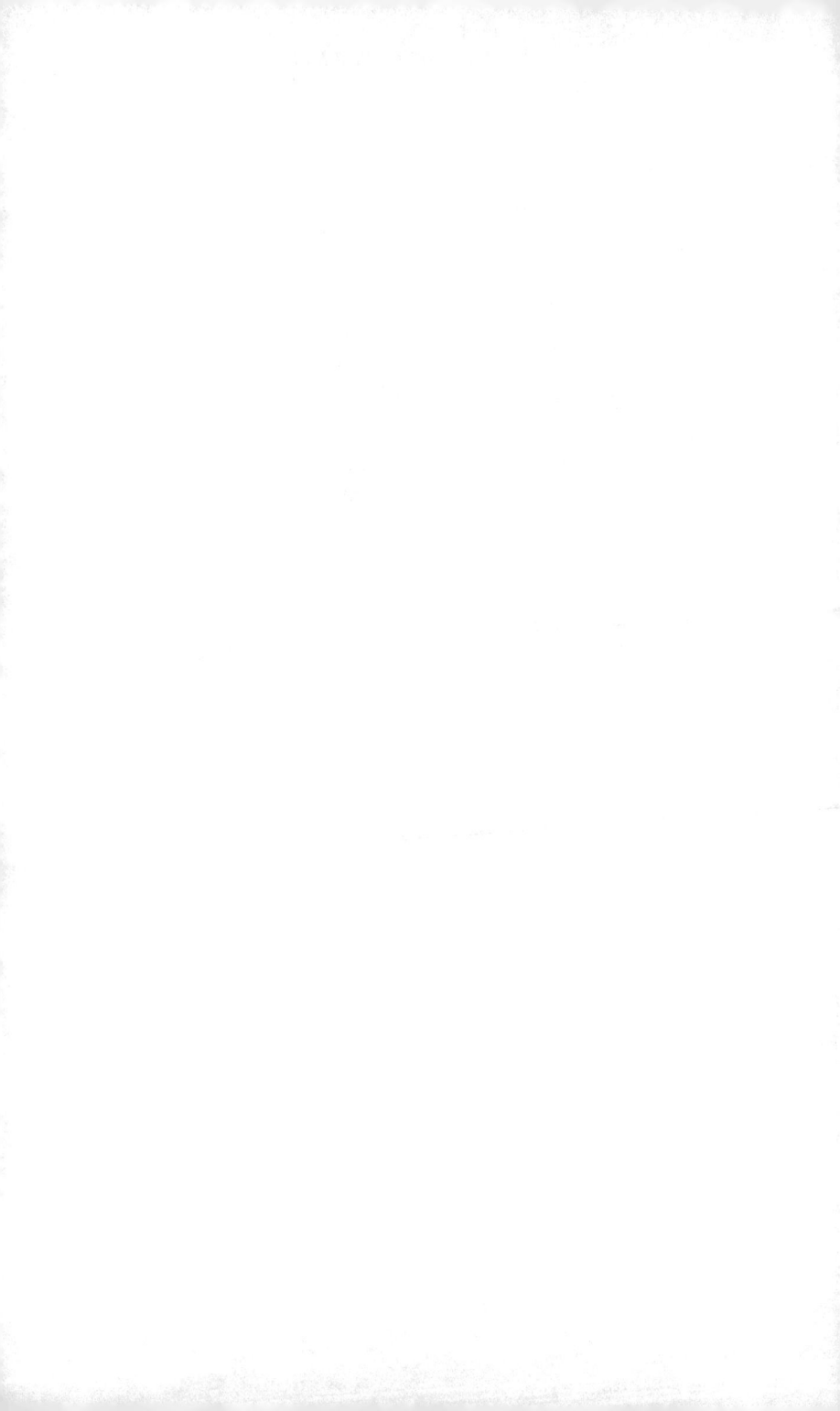